F*CK
INSURANCE

YOUR PLAYBOOK TO A SUCCESSFUL
PERFORMANCE PT PRACTICE AND
NEVER HAVING TO DEAL WITH
INSURANCE AGAIN

DANNY MATTA

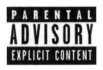

FREE STUFF!

Thanks so much for purchasing this book. Before you begin reading, I have some freebies for you!

In addition to the information already provided in this book, I have created a free roadmap and webinar to help you get started.

You can sign up to get your free roadmap here: https://physicaltherapybiz.com

By signing up, you'll also be notified of any pending book releases or updated content and be first in line for exclusive deals and future book giveaways or other kick-ass promotions. No spam; you have my word.

Immediately after signing up you'll be sent an email with access to the free bonus, so be sure to check your inbox.

–Danny Matta

CONTENTS

FOREWORD

Be careful with the book you're holding in your hands. It contains a dangerous idea.

As I write this, it is officially my tenth anniversary of being completely self-employed. For a decade now, my family and I have been living the life contained in the pages of this book.

Fortunately, hindsight tends to pave over momentous life decisions when they work to your advantage. Time and opportunity make it easier to forget the conversations I had with my parents and in-laws about the obviously poor decision I was making to cut the cord and walk away from my "safe" physio job. Or the late nights. Or sleeping on my table in the office after traveling home from teaching a weekend course, knowing I'd start the next day with my first athlete group at 5:30 a.m. Or the stress my wife and I felt juggling two young daughters, a full-time gig as a senior associate in a big San Francisco law firm, and a "start-up."

If I asked my CEO/wife now if she would go back to the traditional land of "safe," she would laugh out loud and say that we are now both unemployable. A decade of living this side of the fence means that we know too much. We have become comfortable with the constant low-grade pressures and uncertainties that come with working for yourself. We have also become accustomed to owning our own time, completely. Do you remember how much possibility the world contained when you first started grad school? It's like that. And once you've experienced it, you can't go back.

That's pretty much what I told Danny during our debrief after teaching a course for him when he was still a rising superstar physio for the Army. For my own ego, I'd love to pretend that I had some small influence on Danny leaving the Army and starting a small revolution in PT business. Alas, it's simply not true. Danny had already created the model contained in this book. He was already networking, already building referral bases, and already shaping his PT practice to better suit the needs of his patients and athletes, as well as his own needs and desires to become a better practitioner. If you're reading this, the die is already cast. It's too late for you. Danny can see it in you the same way I saw it in him. As we say in our house, "Game recognizes Game." The world is ready for you. You already see it.

Of course, the world wasn't always ready. Think of the chutzpah it took to open an independent practice even fifteen or twenty years ago. Those brilliant physios who were able to, did it without the world of Instagram, Facebook, YouTube, CrossFit, SoulCycle, social networks, pop-up ads, search keywords, Yelp … They were true pioneers, trying to make a brave new world while still serving the old gods. It was a slog. How many of the instructors at my PT school had owned PT clinics and sold them? Quite a few. And I understand, completely. The world wasn't ready. The last decade has begun to change how people think about their health and how they pay for it. And all of that "social/tech/innovation" has meant that if you want to play a different work game, you have to be fluent in a set of skills they did not fully prepare you for in grad school. You have to be ready too.

Look, in the spirit of full disclosure, Danny and I are great friends. We've been working alongside each other for quite a few years now.

And damn him for not writing this book before now. For those of us who decided that the world and PT profession were ready for a new practice model, there was no blueprint. We made the best decisions possible in an uncertain and emergent field. And we sucked at it. Clearly I have a bit of a subversive streak. But I'm not alone. I remember thinking in every single one of my observation hours and clinical affiliations, "I can't wait to see 15–20 patients a day and write notes on my lunch, and I love this hung ceiling, and wow the inter-session HEP adherence rate is so great, and those fluorescent lights make my skin look so great, and yes, these are short arc-quads, and maybe smoking and alcohol consumption and not sleeping and your job stress and the fact you hate your job may have something to do with your back pain, oh and also why is everyone working here so burned out?"

What I'm saying is, you and I and Danny all knew something wasn't right when we started this process. What we also knew in the core of our soul? We were born for this. This book isn't the only way home, but it is a sure thing. Subversive? Even the brilliant thinker Buckminster Fuller knew the only way to make a model obsolete is not to rage from inside the system, but rather to propose a new, better model that makes the old one obsolete. The model that all my friends use is: test, retest, share. This wonderful book follows exactly the scientific model proposed by The Godfather of science, Sir Francis Bacon. Sir Francis Bacon wrote that the heart of science was induction through observation and pattern recognition. Danny has done the heavy lifting for us.

So go ahead, prove his model wrong. Break it. Improve upon it. Make us obsolete. We will be here and ready to follow. Dangerous ideas cannot be contained.

Kelly Starrett, DPT

ACKNOWLEDGMENTS

My mom once told me that everyone has a poem, a painting, and a book inside them. I'm not a good painter, and I don't know the first thing about poetry, but I guess I can check off one of the three with this book.

I also can imagine she didn't expect the book living inside me to be titled *F*ck Insurance*. Either way, thanks for the inspiration, and this one's for you, Mom.

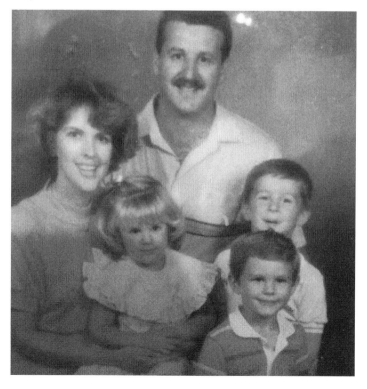

INTRODUCTION

Full disclosure: my wife was not a big fan of the title of this book. In fact, many people will be put off by the title of this book. I realize it may sound a bit extreme, so I want to explain exactly what I mean by "fuck insurance."

First, it's no secret that health insurance companies are huge organizations that frankly don't give a fuck about you. They don't care about you as a consumer or as a practitioner. I realized this personally when I got out of the Army and found myself paying around $1,000 a month for insurance premiums. This was with a $3,500 deductible. A $1,000 premium is a mortgage payment, and it's crazy to think that's what it takes to insure my family. You're talking about people who drink dehydrated greens, look at elaborate blood panels preventively, eat healthy food, and prioritize being active.

We realized insurance wasn't set up for people like us. We are outliers, and we choose to go to the providers we want to see, not who insurance says we can see. Because of that, we get the highest deductible plan we can afford and put the max amount of money into an HSA account. We are informed consumers, and it's our money we're spending on high-quality, outside-the-box-thinking providers.

The reality is, there are a lot of people like us out there. These people are trying to be proactive, not reactive, with their health. These are the people who we predominately see at our practice. It just makes sense for them to spend their money on seeing an expert who can make decisions that are best for them. Insurance has no effect on what we tell someone they need to do or what our plan of care is.

This segment of the population is middle-aged, active, and informed. These are the people who fall through the cracks in a traditional PT setting. These are the fifty-year-old runners trying to continue marathon training for life. These are the thirty-five-year-old dads and moms who want to keep playing in a pick-up soccer league. These are the forty-year-old CrossFitters who are trying to stay in great shape but also stay around their friends at the gym. These middle-aged active "overachievers" are who we work with every day. A mere 3 sets of 10 on the shuttle won't do it for these people. Clamshells won't do it for these people. They require more complexity. They require a Performance Physical Therapist. Many of you would kill to work with people like this every day. The model I show you in this book will get you to that point. Insurance will not allow you to work with people in the capacity you want. Because of that, we have to go outside of insurance.

"Fuck insurance" is also directed toward another group. It's directed toward the corporate-owned, high-volume PT practices that are burning out our brightest young PTs.

I realize there are a lot of privately owned insurance-taking practices out there. I honestly feel bad for these practices because they are just trying to stay in business. They get pushed around by insurance companies. They get paid less and have very little leverage with negotiations. They can either increase the number of people they see or try to sell to some larger clinic that does have more leverage. This group in particular can benefit from this book. Adding more cash-paying patients to your revenue can stabilize your business. Not only that, but you can get back to using your skill set the way it was designed to be used. You can use your hands more. You can solve more complex problems because you actually have the time for it. You can cut down the ridiculous amount of documentation you have to do just to get paid. I hope this book helps you and allows you to get back to loving what you do again.

Now, back to those high-volume, corporate-owned PT mills. I want them to see what's happening. When you take a motivated young PT and throw 20–40 people on their schedule in a day, that's wrong. They know it's wrong, and they're doing it because it's profitable. In the process, they're burning out the people who are supposed to lead our profession one day. Just look at the movement of the non-clinical PT. These PTs are searching for ways to transfer their experience over to other professions. Some of them go back and become financial planners, accountants, or managers in corporate environments.

When I see this trend, here's what I want to know: Do you really not want to be a PT anymore, or do you not want to be a PT in a high-volume setting?

I get it. I've worked in high-volume settings. I've had friends that hung in there at clinics seeing 30–40 people a day with just one tech to help for a year. I saw my same friend's health deteriorate and his love for his profession disappear; eventually, he moved on to doing home health PT. He didn't do this because he loved home health work. He did this because he made more and worked less. He did this because he didn't have any other option.

Do you think these PT mills feel bad about that? Fuck no they don't. Many of them are owned by private equity firms or hospital organizations. These people care more about what their profit and loss sheet shows than the happiness of their employees. I'm all for a profitable business, but not at the expense of the future of our profession.

So to the PT mills and the insurance companies, I say, "Fuck you." I say this for the thousands of underpaid and overworked PTs you employ right now. In this profession, we are tired of you forcing us into roles that lead us to question if we should have even gone to PT school in the first place. This book will arm this group of PTs fed up with your bullshit with another option. An option to take their careers back into their own hands. An option to break away from the unsustainable career path they are currently on. An option to make more money and have more time with their friends and families. An option to get back to loving what they do. An option to truly help people and develop long-term relationships. In particular, an option for these Performance PTs to use their skill sets to change our healthcare landscape forever.

This is an exciting time to be a PT. Too many people are down on our profession. They just can't see what's actually happening. They can't see the revolution that's taking place. They can't see the potential we have and how much we can do for the people around us. This book will open your eyes. It will help you realize that you are part of this revolution, and you should be proud of that.

That's it. The line in the sand has been drawn. You have to pick a side. You can continue with the status quo and be a sheep force-fed an endless number of patients all day. Step across that line and become one of us. You can be a wolf that goes out and gets what you want in life. You can make your degree work for you in whatever capacity that is. You can build a business that allows you to love what you do for a living and create financial freedom at the same time.

Now it's up to you. You have to choose. You can't live in the middle, straddling the line. Do you want to be a sheep, or do you want to be a wolf?

I want to take a deep dive into different phases of building a

Performance Cash PT Clinic because many of you will fall into one of these phases. If you're just starting out, it can be difficult to think about getting to the point in your business where you have employees. But that shouldn't be the focus right out of the gate. In the beginning, just focus on getting to the next phase.

Each phase has different obstacles and revenue ranges. Focus on going from phase 1 to phase 2. Don't focus on going from phase 1 to phase 5.

My son trains Jiu Jitsu, and he is a white belt. He practices, learns submissions, grapples, and has some fun. He has a goal of getting a black belt one day. In Jiu Jitsu, this could take ten to twelve years. I don't think as many people would stick around if one day, ten years from the time they started, they just got handed a black belt. There's a stripe and belt system that keeps people motivated along the way. Think of the phases I lay out as belts. When you get from phase 1 to 2, celebrate. It's like getting a blue belt in Jiu Jitsu. Then get back to work and start trying to get from phase 2 to phase 3.

My goal is for you to have a profitable seven-figure business that you love being part of and that impacts people in a very positive way. Starting our business has done amazing things for my family. I hope this book helps you achieve the same results.

SECTION 1:

THE FIVE PHASES OF THE CASH PERFORMANCE PT CLINIC

CHAPTER 1

MY STORY AND HOW WE GOT TO THIS POINT

I remember sitting in my driveway in September of 2013. It was no different than any other morning during the workweek. I was about to leave to head in to my assignment at Ft. Benning. At the time, I was working at a Troop Medical Clinic attached to the US Army Airborne School. We had sick call hours that started around 6 a.m., so I had been up since about 4:30.

Normally, I just got in my car, started an audiobook, and drove into work. That morning, however, I got in my car and just sat there. I sat there and physically didn't want to turn the key to start the car. I dreaded driving to work. It was the first time in my career that I felt like I didn't want to be a physical therapist anymore.

I had recently left the job of my dreams, and I hadn't yet recovered from the loss.

In my last job, I had been assigned to work as a Brigade Physical Therapist for 2nd Brigade in the 25th Infantry Division. When I first got there, very few people knew why they had been assigned a PT, let alone what I actually did.

The first six months or so in the job were really difficult. I had a huge backlog of injured soldiers that needed to be seen. I also had to work at trying to educate everyone on how I could help them.

Because they knew very little about me or what I was supposed to do, I had almost no guidance or supervision. This was actually not a bad thing for me, and I thrived in that situation. I knew I needed to leverage my skill set somehow because our brigade had about 4,000 soldiers. One PT for 4,000 soldiers is a very difficult task.

I eventually ended up developing systems for a few medics I was given to help me. These injury protocols and systems allowed me to cut my patient treatment time in half. I got to teach more proactive movement classes and strength/conditioning classes, and I started helping improve the physical training of the brigade.

They gave me an office in the common area of some barracks, right between a laundromat and the rec room, which had a TV plus foosball and ping pong tables. The best part of this location was that on the second floor of this building was a fully built out gym called the Sweat Factory!

Most of my work with this brigade took place in the Sweat Factory. The gym was laid out like a big CrossFit gym, a combatives area taking up about a third of the space. I could take groups or individuals up to the gym and go over any movement you could imagine. The more I taught people how to move well and take care of themselves, the fewer injuries I saw. Not only that, but those same soldiers also started performing better at physical events they had previously struggled with.

This situation was a dream come true for me. I was now functioning as a Performance Physical Therapist. I was living in the gray area between rehab and performance training. I got to teach strength/conditioning class, work on injury prevention programs, and treat soldiers. It gave me a lot of options, and I loved this time in my career.

These were my guys, and we were all training for the common goal of being ready to go when we deployed in August of 2013. We were on the books to head out to Kandahar, Afghanistan, for twelve months. It was like a really big sports team training together for some long-term crucible event with real-life consequences. I knew the healthier we could get and keep our soldiers, the more likely it was they could be successful at their jobs.

In April of 2013, I took part in our very last brigade-wide training event. At these events, the entire brigade participated in coordinated training together. Think of it like a really big scrimmage. The infantry guys went out on simulated missions; the communication elements made sure all of their radios and gear were working, and the medical providers set up a massive tent hospital.

In this situation, I had my own section of the tent for my treatment office. It was connected to the dental section. The dentist and I both had additional roles. He was the main triage officer, and I was the second. This basically meant that if a massive casualty situation were to happen, he and I decided who got help and who was in such bad shape they probably wouldn't make it. This was a massive responsibility, and we took our training very seriously even though neither of us had trauma experience.

On the last day of this final brigade-wide event, I was sitting in the dental clinic going over trauma triage protocols with our brigade dentist. I felt my phone buzz in my pocket and looked at it. It was a text message from LTC Honeycutt, our direct battalion commander. This meant he was in charge of about 600 of us. I had never gotten a text message from him before. The message was simple, and I'll never forget it: "Deployment canceled, have a nice weekend. LTC Honeycutt."

To say this left me confused and frustrated is an understatement. I had spent the last year and a half training for a deployment to Afghanistan. And it was called off with one text message. Very little explanation was given as to why this happened except that our role had to be changed to Pacific Region development.

My wife, Ashley, was four months pregnant with our daughter, Maggie, at the time. In many ways, this was a huge blessing. First, I wouldn't have to miss her birth and leave Ashley by herself to care for two young kids while I was gone in a hostile country for a year.

I also know in some respects this spared me from going through the life-altering experiences that are so commonly seen in deployed environments. Many of my friends had come back different people, including my brother, who had spent fifteen months working as a nurse in a Baghdad emergency room years before.

At the same time, I was mad. I was mad that I had volunteered for this and trained for this; now I felt robbed of the experience. I wanted to do my job in an environment that would absolutely test my skills. I selfishly wanted to know how I would react in real-life dangerous situations, not simulated ones. It's hard to describe because it was both a positive and a negative time in my life.

I spent the next few weeks talking to our human resources director, trying to figure out what was next in my military career. At the same time, I had been offered an opportunity from Kelly Starrett. He was someone who was leading the charge for Performance PTs. His book *Becoming a Supple Leopard* had recently become a best seller, and there was literally no person on the planet I would rather have had the opportunity to work with. He was expanding his team of instructors and had asked me if I was interested in joining the team. Of course I said yes, but I still wasn't sure if that meant I would leave the Army entirely or just teach for them on the side.

Regardless, my time with the 25th Infantry Division had come to an end. I was usually reassigned to a new post every three years, and the three-year mark on my current assignment was closing in.

Once I was reassigned to Ft. Benning, everything changed. No longer did I have the autonomy I loved so much. No longer did I have the ability to work as a Performance PT and function in this hybrid strength/PT role. I was placed back in a traditional clinic position. My volume was relatively high because we had so many people coming in for sick call. I felt like a cog in a wheel, and I hated it.

After about ten minutes of sitting there in my car that morning and thinking about how resistant I was to driving to work, I finally got going. The audiobook I listened to was *To Sell Is Human* by Daniel Pink. As I listened to the book, I thought about my options:

Option 1: I could stay in the Army, continue to get promoted, and retire with a pension and full healthcare for life in just thirteen more years. My dad and both of my grandfathers had chosen this option. It had always seemed like the most logical thing to do.

Option 2: I could get out of the Army and try to make something work on my own.

To make things even more stressful, Ashley was due to have Maggie in about a month. Talk about the wrong time to have reservations about your current career path.

I was totally distracted thinking about these options all day. Over lunch I had a conversation with one of the other PTs, Jeremy Houser. He was very entrepreneurial and had become a good friend of mine. He made it seem like a no-brainer: get out of the Army, go into practice for myself, and try to do things differently than the traditional PT model. He said, "Fuck insurance. People will pay to work with you one-on-one no matter if insurance covers it or not."

After the excitement of my conversation with Jeremy wore off, I went back and forth for weeks about what I actually wanted to do. I talked with Ashley, and she was supportive of whatever choice I wanted to pursue.

What really pushed me to leave the Army and start my own business was a conversation I had with one of my patients. He was an Airborne instructor retiring from the Army after twenty years of service.

He and I chatted about his plans for retirement. He was so excited to talk about it. He lit up like a Christmas tree telling me about how he was going to start his own photography business. He said, "I've always loved photography and am so excited to start a business where I can do what I love every day."

I asked him if he felt that way about being in the Army. He laughed a little bit and said, "I haven't loved what I do in the Army for about ten years." He explained that as he got higher ranks, he started to do more and more tasks he hated. The only reason he'd stuck with it for the last ten years was because he wanted the pension and healthcare retirement. He felt staying in the Army was the "safe" choice.

That was it. I didn't want to look back at my career and be okay with making the "safe" choice. I didn't want to look forward to starting my own businesses for the next thirteen years if I stayed in the Army. I wanted to put all my eggs in one basket, my own basket, and bet on myself.

I finished the next eight months in the Army then separated from active duty in June of 2014. I started Athletes' Potential that same month.

I found an office to sublease in a CrossFit gym in West Atlanta. That office was in the corner of a gym. It had no windows. It was the bare minimum I needed to start a company and a movement in the city.

I was terrified and excited at the same time. I was back to being able to function in the Performance PT role I enjoyed so much. I was taking my career and future into my own hands. I had no idea what

I was doing. I did have a family to support, and that's about all the motivation you need to work hard every day.

I did it on a shoestring budget: massage table from Costco (who doesn't love Costco?), desk and chairs from Ikea, and just enough equipment to be able to see people effectively.

For under $3,000, I started my practice. I didn't have to take a loan or max out my credit cards.

I honestly knew very little about business, and I moved to a city where I was new, which meant no one knew who I was or what I could do.

There was one thing I knew I could do. I could teach and educate the masses. And that's exactly what I did from day one. For the next six months I taught about movement, mobility, strength, and self-treatment one to two times a week. I've taught in every type of gym you can imagine. I've taught at small businesses, tech companies, consulting firms, government offices, and even in a florist shop.

Within six months, I went from zero people on my schedule to twenty patient visits per week, charging $175 a visit. These were all cash-based visits, and I didn't deal with a single insurance company.

Fast forward four years later. We have grown to a standalone, 2,000 square-foot facility and one satellite office in a gym. We have four full-time PTs and an amazing administrative staff. We work with our patients on our terms. We spend more time with and develop stronger relationships with our patients than any clinic in the city.

None of this, by the way, would have been possible without my extremely talented wife, Ashley. She is the integrator that holds Athletes' Potential together. She's a badass who doesn't take shit from people, and she keeps the business highly organized. Having talent like her on our team has been vital to our company. If it wasn't for her, I'd probably still be seeing people in that windowless room in the corner of a dirty gym.

During these past four years, I've grown tremendously as a clinician, businessman, parent, spouse, and human being. The process has been challenging, stressful, exciting, terrifying, rewarding, and fun as hell—all at the same time.

Starting a business and having children are the scariest and most rewarding things I've done in my life. I hope you decide to bet on yourself like I did.

In this book I hope to shed some light on the lessons we've learned and how you can apply them to your business. More importantly, I strongly believe in the power of the Performance PT model. We have such a unique skill set, and it gets watered down by high-volume PT mill-style clinics. These clinics are burning out our best young PTs with massive volume, poor pay, and an endless number of patients they have very little interest in working with. They focus more on revenue than the people in their company or the patients that walk through their doors. If you're a Performance PT, you're a Ferrari! Putting a Ferrari in a PT mill is like driving a Ferrari only through school zones. You can only drive that sucker 25 miles an hour for so long before you get frustrated and really want to test out what it can do.

I was once told that if you can't find the job of your dreams, you have to create it. Our current landscape doesn't allow for many people to work in this low-volume, one-on-one setting. If you can't find a position like this, you have to create it yourself.

Talented PTs like you can not only get people out of pain but also teach them how to squat, run, swim, and move their bodies better. You could specialize in golf, tennis, CrossFit, triathlons, or whatever other movement discipline you're interested in. Your unique ability to live in the gray area between performance and rehab is where we can help people the most.

The more of us who have successful practices, the more people we help, and the stronger the profession becomes. More of us growing our business to multiple providers allows us to have great jobs for those providers who have no interest in entrepreneurship. There are a lot of great Performance PTs out there looking to work in a setting like this as well.

We are in the middle of a Performance PT revolution.

Even though we all know clinical skills are vital, if you do not understand the basics of business, you will always struggle with success.

Doesn't it make you mad that the clinician down the street is always packed while you keep having to help fix patients he/she can't get better? Well, that clinician may not be able to hold a candle to your clinical skills, but they might be way better at sales and marketing. These skills are just as vital to the health of your business as your clinical skills; they are so important to understand.

This book will sharpen your business skills and empower you to help even more people in your area. This is the roadmap to financial and time freedom that I have found through starting a cash physical therapy practice.

This is your roadmap. It's not the easy road, but if you stay the course, you will find success. You'll get out of the rat race and become not just a successful PT but a successful entrepreneur.

You cannot dream yourself into a character; you must hammer and forge yourself one.

—James A. Froude

CHAPTER 2

FROM FRUSTRATION TO EPIPHANY

I was once told that starting a business is kind of like throwing up. We've all been there. Maybe you caught a little stomach bug, or maybe you drank too much one night. You have that queasy feeling in your stomach. You don't want to puke, but you know that if you do, afterward you'll feel a lot better. That's how I felt when I was on the fence about starting my own business. When I finally decided to do it, I had a lot of discomfort—like I was just waiting to throw up. Once I got through that initial discomfort, I felt relieved and so much better about my professional career going forward.

After I decided to start my own practice, the questions really came down to one major question: *Insurance or no insurance?*

After doing some research and talking to colleagues, I realized I was not well equipped to play the insurance game. I just hated the idea that I would be reimbursed for certain things but not others. I didn't want a third party telling me what I should and shouldn't do with my patients.

Like many of you, I find this is one of the most frustrating parts of working for or owning an in-network practice. The real question was: *If I don't take insurance, will it work?*

I was fortunate enough to have a good relationship with my mentor, Kelly Starrett. He had started a cash PT practice in San Francisco about four years before I decided to start my business. I knew he was treating people on a cash basis, with minimal equipment and had a waitlist to get in to see him. He recommended I think about my perfect patient—the patient I looked forward to working with every day. Then, he said, build a practice that catered exactly to that group. This way I'd have a unique bond with my patients and I'd get more fulfillment and energy out of working with these people.

I knew I wanted to work with young, active, and highly motivated people.

I also thought back to my previous career as a personal trainer, before going to Physical Therapy school. I knew way less at that point in my life and had people paying me $80 a session 2–3 times a week for personal training. I really enjoyed the one-on-one relationship and connection I had with my clients.

I took Kelly's advice and thought about my dream practice. I want you to do the same thing.

What do you want your practice to look like?
Who do you want to work with?
How do you want it to feel?
How much money do you want to make?
What do you want to never deal with again?
What would a perfect workday look like for you?
How do you want other people to view what you do?

Answer these questions and see if what you're currently doing matches up with your answers. If it doesn't, it's time to make a change. If it does, every day at work will feel like a day off.

The other thing I want you to realize is that many professions have hourly cash rates. No one thinks twice about dropping money on some of these professions. They provide value to people and have a specialized skill set. Take a look:

Dentists
Psychologists

Functional Medicine Providers
Accountants
Lawyers
Engineers
Massage Therapists
Fee-Only Financial Planners
Trainers
Coaches

I thought that if these professions can make a time-based cash service work, I can totally do it too.

Many of us contemplating a cash practice have self-doubt, worrying that people won't pay for our help. We struggle with the mindset shift necessary to move from being an in-network provider to a cash PT business owner. We'll talk more about this in the mindset chapter.

Confidence can get you a long way in life. It's no different in business, and the more you realize there are other successful cash PT owners, the more confidence you should have.

Confidence will naturally build as you ascend through the phases of a gym cash practice.

Everyone starting a business is self-employed. That means you're the owner, PT, administrative director, marketing director, sales director, web developer, and social media director. You're doing everything, and it will always be that way when you first start out.

Here's what I want you to keep in mind. You don't want to *stay* self-employed if you choose to start your own business. A business is not a business unless it functions without you. If it doesn't function without you, it's a job and you're still self-employed.

In these next two chapters, we'll go over two popular strategies to getting started. Getting started is the hardest part, and these two chapters will shed some light on how you can do it.

CHAPTER 3

THE BURN THE SHIPS METHOD

I remember my first day in my cash practice. It was a Monday, and I had literally gotten out of the Army three days before. People told me to take a break and enjoy some time off after I left the Army. I told them I had a wife, a son, and a daughter. I had to pay my mortgage and put food on the table. Taking a break just wasn't an option. The reality is: when you first start your practice, you will be in the survival phase.

There are two different approaches when starting out. You can use the Burn the Ships method or the Side Hustle method.

Let's start with the Burn the Ships method.

In 1519 Captain Hernán Cortés landed in Veracruz, Mexico, with 600 men. After landing, he gave the order to burn all the ships. This sent a very clear message to his men: There is no turning back. There is no quitting. It's either success or death. Two years later he succeeded in his conquest of the Aztec Empire.

We are long past the days of conquering other empires, and as practitioners we're better suited to helping people with their back pain anyway. Still, we can learn a lot from Cortés in regard to his methods of accomplishing his goal.

The Burn the Ships method is the option I chose when starting my practice. I had a bit of a unique circumstance that allowed me to do this.

When I got out of the Army, I had what's called terminal leave. *Terminal leave* refers to the unused vacation days you have accrued while on active duty in the Army. For three of the last four years that I was in the Army I was stationed in Hawaii. I literally lived on a tropical island where people travel long distances to vacation. Needless to say, I didn't use a lot of vacation days. Every day was a vacation!

Because of this, I had almost fifty-eight days of vacation saved. That means I had fifty-eight days of pay, as if I were still in the Army. That also included fifty-eight days of healthcare coverage for my family.

When I decided to burn the ships, my goal was to replace my salary from the Army in fifty-eight days. This was a very aggressive goal, and I felt the only way to accomplish it was to go all in.

Let me stress that this option is not the right option for everyone. I've literally never been more stressed, scared, and unsure of my ability to provide for my family than during those weeks. In particular, having two small kids and starting a new business is a difficult decision no matter what your business is.

That being said, I feel this method is the best way to achieve success as fast as possible. This method made me take a really hard look at my numbers and set a specific goal to achieve in the first two months.

My take-home pay from the Army after taxes was about $5,500 a month. Assuming a 30% tax on what I would currently be making in private practice, I needed to make $7,150 a month to completely offset that salary.

I did some basic math to figure out how many patients I needed to see. I was charging $175 a visit at that time. Divide that $7,150 by my per-visit rate, and we're talking about forty patients.

I would have to see forty patients to make the same amount I was getting paid *and* make the transition relatively smooth on our family.

When I broke it down even further, I started to gain some confidence that I could actually pull this off.

Forty patients in a month meant I basically needed to reach ten visits a week. That was just two patients a day if I had a five-day-a-week schedule. Two patients a day? Seriously, I was used to seeing over twenty a day. How hard could two patients a day be?

Well, it's actually really hard. If you've already started a practice, you know those first few months can be tough on your confidence. Adversity leads many people to stay in their office and just hope that things will work out. Here's my advice if you're in that self-destructive part of starting your business: Get the fuck out of your little office and go meet people. It's not how many people you know, it's how many people know you.

This is exactly what I did. In those first two months, I set up teaching events one or two nights a week. I conducted about a dozen teaching events at gyms around the area in the first two months. On average, I got 1–3 new patients right away every time I taught. That meant by the end of the first two months I had already generated about twenty new patients.

I had twenty-two visits the first month. I had thirty-five visits the second month. And by the third month, I was up to fifty visits. This allowed me to replace the salary I had been getting in the Army dollar for dollar and keep food on the table for the kiddos! Luckily for us, they love mac and cheese; that shit is cheap.

When you burn the ships and set an aggressive goal, you give yourself no other alternative.

I like to play this game with my brother-in-law where I ask him ridiculous questions and see how much money I would have to pay him to get him to try things. I'll say, "Brandon, if I gave you a parachute, how much money would I have to pay you to jump off the tallest building in Atlanta?" We then proceed to negotiate this hypothetical event and the money needed to do this task.

One time I asked him how much I would have to give him to run a 100-mile race. We settled on our hypothetical amount. Then I asked him: if his daughter Emery were in trouble 100 miles away and he had to run there, would he run it faster? He got very serious and said, "Absolutely. And I'd run as fast and as far as I physically could if she needed me."

When you burn the ships and have family counting on you, you'll push as fast and far as you physically can in order to provide for them. My family was my motivation. The other important factor to keep in mind is that you have to be *completely committed* to achieving this goal.

I recently had the opportunity to talk to the third-year Indiana State University Doctorate of Physical Therapy students. This interview was set up by someone who's already come up once in this book, Jeremy Houser. After we both left the clinic where we worked in Columbus, he went on to get his PhD. Now he's a professor at Indiana State, and he asked me to talk to his students about entrepreneurship. I love talking to students, so I jumped at the chance.

I fielded the normal questions about how to get patients, which continuing education courses to attend, and marketing through social media. Toward the end of the Q&A, a student raised a question I had never encountered before. He asked, "If your business isn't doing well, how do you know when it's time to give up?" Almost reflexively, I said, "Never." I quickly realized that was a bit of a jackass answer, so I explained what I meant by that.

Here's what I explained—I'm sharing it with you because I think it's the most important part of this book. If you're like me, constantly skimming text for key points, don't do that with this chapter.

In order to be successful in something as difficult as starting and growing a thriving business, you have to be *fully committed to the result*. Not only that—you have to take full ownership of the result before you start or learn how to do all the things you need to do to be successful.

I'm NOT talking about just visualizing success in your mind every night while you're drinking some special tea that's supposed to help with cognitive function. Take that bullshit tea and dump it down the drain where it belongs. I mean you have to take 100% ownership of the fact that <u>you are going to make this thing work</u>.

I've had plenty of setbacks in business, and I've made a lot of mistakes. I'm sure I'll make more mistakes in the future; I'll have difficult events or scenarios surface. I accept that, and I am absolutely willing to deal with whatever those things are. I have committed to the goal of building this company, and nothing is going to stop that—not you, not a competitor, not the government, not fear, and not rejection. I could lose every dollar I have tomorrow, and I would still continue to work on achieving this goal.

When I first started Athletes' Potential, it wasn't unusual for me to put in 60+ hours a week and then travel two to three times a month to teach for Kelly Starrett's group, MobilityWOD. I would teach from 8 a.m. until 6 p.m. Saturday and Sunday. Then I'd jump on a flight and head right back to Atlanta to get back to work at home. It's not an exaggeration when I say I worked 300+ hours a month, and I worked at this clip for almost two years.

During those first two years, my health suffered, and so did my relationship with my wife, Ashley. I was in the worst shape of my life, I was temperamental, and I wasn't the most enjoyable person to be around. Honestly, I was tired, but I was so hyper-focused on succeeding that I continued to push myself.

When I get a question like that—When do you know when it's time to give up?—I think about those first two years. It would have been so easy to give up. I could have stopped and gotten a good-paying job at any number of places in Atlanta. I could have started playing sports again and spent more time with Ashley. It would have been the easy solution, but I knew it would eat me up inside if I did that. There was no other option. I had already taken ownership of the fact that I had to see this through.

I'm not telling you that you should sacrifice your health and relationships with your loved ones for success in business. I *am* saying that great things do not come easily. If it were easy, why wouldn't everyone play in the NFL? Why wouldn't everyone climb Mt. Everest? Why wouldn't everyone have a successful business of their own?

Very few people do these things because they are difficult. They require sacrifice and effort. Not just for a day or a week but for years and even decades.

Tony Robbins once said, "Most people overestimate what they can do in a year and they underestimate what they can do in two or three decades."[1] This is such an accurate statement, and the long-term commitment is what stops most people from achieving success.

I'm not here to sugarcoat this and tell you this is going to be easy and you'll make hundreds of thousands of dollars next year. That's just not reality. If reading this chapter is enough to make you rethink going into business for yourself, good. You would have given up anyway.

---

1   *Tony Robbins: I Am Not Your Guru*, directed by Joe Berlinger, 2016, on Netflix, https://core.tonyrobbins.com/documentary/.

If reading this chapter motivates you and excites you to take on one of the greatest challenges in life, good. You're the one who can benefit from the rest of this book. You're the one who, when someone asks when to give up, you immediately respond, "Never." You're the one who will put in the work and the sacrifice, the one who will take the pain. You're the one who will look back years from now and realize you've been able to create something other people only dream about. You'll have financial freedom, and your family's lives will change for generations. You'll have time freedom and live a life on your terms. You'll be one of the few who get to experience the world in a special, unique way.

It all starts with a commitment. A real, true, deeply rooted internal commitment to achieve what you're setting out to accomplish. If you can't do that, the Burn the Ships strategy is not the right strategy for you.

CHAPTER 4

THE SIDE HUSTLE METHOD

For many people, burning the ships sounds extremely stressful and makes them want to vomit. Don't worry, it's not the only way. There is another, less stressful but still effect method, the Side Hustle method.

There are a few different ways to do a side hustle practice that I'll go into. All of them share a common theme of starting a business while still working another job. This way you don't cut off all the money you're making at once. I'll give you two examples of members of my mastermind group that started their practices with this method.

The first member left his full-time outpatient ortho job and took a PRN position that also had health benefits. This is a perfect option if you can find something similar. It wasn't the work he wanted to do for the rest of his life, but it was the perfect job to support him as he set up his side hustle. He worked Tuesday, Wednesday, and Saturday of every week. He made about 70% of what he made while he was full time in his outpatient job, and he got health benefits.

This was really important because he had a wife and two young children.

Once he was able to make enough to replace his full-time salary with his gym practice, he stopped working for the PRN company.

He basically worked two jobs and put a ton of time in while building his practice. There's no way around that. You will have to work hard; you'll have to get in front of people, network, market, hustle, and be a great practitioner no matter what option you choose.

The other member of my mastermind group took a different approach to starting his side hustle. He is a really good strength coach and worked with clients as a personal trainer while going through PT school. He started to get very busy with school and decided he would only be able to do online programming for his clients; he would have to give up in-person work.

This actually worked out really well for him because he could do the work on his time, and it was all digital. He started charging about $200 a month for individualized programs for his clients. He had about fifteen clients as he finished his last year of school. He built that up to about twenty-five clients his first year out of PT school and set up a really nice side revenue stream for himself.

When he decided to open a cash practice in a gym, he was already making about $5,000 a month doing programming. That's a really nice way to supplement your new venture into a private practice without burning the ships.

These two examples have a few things in common. They both started with a smaller but stable revenue stream before jumping into building a practice. These side jobs offered the flexibility to build relationships and their business during the week. They both successfully implemented a side hustle method and now have standalone cash PT practices in gyms.

There are countless other variations of the side hustle start. I do, however, want you to think about the power of the digital programming business example. This man was one of the first people I coached who was doing a significant amount of individualized programming. This approach has become much more popular over the past few years. People will pay $150–$350 a month for individualized programming to follow. This requires no direct in-person time and can be done from anywhere. It can even be done while you are in school (yes, I'm talking to you, students). We'll get into more on the digital business arena later, but let that little mind bomb soak in for a minute.

In the next few chapters I am going to take you through the phases of the Gym PT Model.

Below is the Gym PT Success Pyramid. Wherever you currently find yourself on this pyramid, your goal should be to get your business to the top of that pyramid.

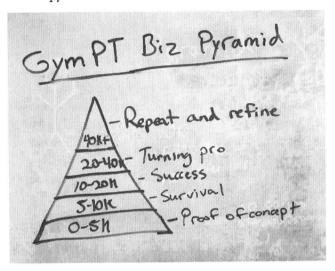

Understanding where you are and what you need to focus on is half the battle! Let's get to it.

Phase 1—Proof of concept: 0–5K in monthly revenue

Phase 2—Survival: 5–10K in monthly revenue

Phase 3—Success: 10–20K in monthly revenue

Phase 4—Turning pro and building a team: 20–40K in monthly revenue

Phase 5—Repeat and refine: 40K+ in monthly revenue

CHAPTER 5

PROOF OF CONCEPT PHASE: 0–5K IN MONTHLY REVENUE

Phase 1 for a Gym PT is all about the struggle. One helpful book you might want to pick up and read is *The Dip by Seth Godin*. I know, you're probably saying to yourself, "Seriously, Danny, I'm already reading this book. Now I have to go get another one?" I know, this can feel like book overload, but periodically throughout this book, I'll recommend others. I'm a huge fan of books and how impactful they can be on your journey as an entrepreneur. *The Dip* will help you get comfortable with being uncomfortable. It's also super short and has pictures! That's my kind of book.

Look, you can't start a business and expect it to be smooth sailing the entire time. The start of your business is honestly the most exciting time. It's the reason why so many entrepreneurs start multiple businesses. They are excited by the potential. They are excited by the opportunity and the chance to build something great. It will also feel like you're pushing a prowler with five of your friends sitting on it. These friends will also be yelling at you about what a bad idea it is to start your own practice and not take insurance. Your friends don't know shit; keep pushing that prowler!

The start is hard; if it weren't, everyone would do it. Get your mind right because you're going to doubt yourself, and your friends and family are going to have reservations about what you're doing, and you're going to get turned down a lot in the beginning.

Now, back to that prowler with your friends sitting on it. This phase is tough, but the excitement will get you through it. You did it. You started your company and now have a business card that says Name, CEO/Founder/Total Badass on it! Enjoy this moment because it is special. Very few of your peers will ever take this step. Congratulations!

Once the joy of becoming an entrepreneur wears off, you'll probably be scared shitless. Here are a few questions you'll be asking yourself during this first phase.

Why did I do this?
What if no one works with me?
What will my family think if I can't make it work?
Am I going to ruin myself financially if I can't make this work?
What if I can't get someone's injury better?
Maybe I'm charging too much. Should I charge less?

These questions ran through my mind countless times in that first phase. My best advice to you is: *Know* these questions will come. But *don't* focus on them. Focus on the processes and the work that needs to be done.

Here's the main goal for this first phase: Get the first 25–50 people in your door and show them what a badass practitioner you are. Give them the best healthcare experience they've ever had, and ask them if they have any friends or family members they think would benefit from your help.

This short pitch, said correctly and with actual sincerity, can change your business:

> Hey, [insert patient name], I just wanted to thank you for coming in to work with me. It's amazing to see the changes you've been able to make and the activities you've been able to get back to.
>
> If you don't mind, I'd love to ask a favor of you. We are a small business, and because of that, we don't have huge marketing

budgets like other corporate-owned PT clinics. Most of our business is driven by word-of-mouth referrals from clients just like you.

If you know anyone like you, who has been dealing with a frustrating and lingering pain/problem, I would greatly appreciate it if you would pass my name along to them.

Seriously, if you take nothing else away from this book, remember the pitch you just read. Your patients will get to know you in this model. They will root for you and want you to succeed. They also love getting a personal win by helping out a friend. You just have to ask them to help you—in an honest and transparent way. Too many PTs I coach or do business consulting with forget this one simple opportunity to ask patients to help them get more patients.

This phase is also the perfect time to look for key coaching staff, trainers, and gym owners. The best way to make connections with these people is to offer them a few free sessions. This allows for several things to happen: First, it gets them familiar with your process so they can tell others in detail about what you do. It also allows you to show off to a person who is influential with your target audience. These key relationships will help drive the right people to you early on.

The other essential aspect of this phase is to use these influential relationships to help connect you with other key relationships. Cold calling is tough. Cold emailing is even worse. Getting someone to introduce you to a potential key relationship will help you out significantly. These warm introductions give you credibility and will dramatically improve your likelihood of developing a solid business relationship with this new person.

Lastly, you have to get out and show people your personality. It's not enough to get out and do workshops so people realize how smart you are. There are a lot of smart people, but clients do business with people they like. Getting teaching events/workshops set up in your local community is a HUGE driver of new business. These events have to be fun and memorable for you to actually get new patients from them. People will come for the knowledge, but they'll work with you because of your personality. Workshops are something we'll take a deep dive on later in this book.

CHAPTER 6

SURVIVAL PHASE: 5–10K IN MONTHLY REVENUE

It's funny when you look back fondly on difficult things you have done in life.

I remember hating summer football practices when I was in high school. One year in particular my dad was reassigned to an Army post in Columbus, Georgia. Columbus is lovingly nicknamed the "Armpit of Georgia." During football practices in the summer, lasting three to four hours, I definitely felt like I was running around in full pads in someone's sweaty armpit.

That summer, my dad went out of his way to get my brother and me jobs we would "love."

This was a common strategy with my dad. Every job he helped us get seemed to involve manual labor and working around people who had pretty hard lives.

My job that summer was detailing cars at the famous Goo Goo Car Wash. We would show up at 7:30 a.m. and proceed to dry, polish, and detail the heck out of whatever cars came through that day. We did this while the owner of the car sat in a lawn chair next to a fan, pointing out all the spots we missed and telling us what a bad job we were doing. It didn't usually get bad until about 9 a.m.—that's when it really started getting hot. Sitting inside cars, spraying chemicals on the leather to condition it, I was drenched in sweat. I quickly realized this was not the life for me.

We would get a 45-minute lunch break every day and then were back to work until about three o'clock. Football practice started at four, so we had about an hour to do nothing. This usually entailed us driving up to the weight room and napping on a bench. We would throw our pads on and head out to practice or passing league until about seven or eight in the evening.

We'd head home, take a shower, and pass out.

We woke up the next morning and started it all over again.

This was how we spent our summer. As exhausting as it was, my brother and I often talk about that time with fond memories.

We have hilarious stories about the characters we worked with. We also got exposed to a group of people who had really hard lives. It gave us an appreciation for difficult work and a strong desire to make a living some other way.

We also bonded that summer more than any other. We were in it together, and it sucked for both of us. Misery loves company, I guess. For as much work as that was, life was simple; and, in some ways, we miss that experience.

It drives me crazy when I hear people say they don't want to do something because it's too much work. Nothing worth doing is ever too much work.

Starting your practice is going to be too much work. You're going to wonder why you decided to do this in the first place. But you'll get past that difficult part, and your practice *will* succeed. Don't be surprised if you look back on those difficult times with fond memories.

You'll find purpose and pride in knowing that what you're doing is not something everyone can do. You are resilient, and you'll find out just how resilient you are once you go into business for yourself.

Also, remember this: If you fail and give up, you might just end up at the Goo Goo Car Wash detailing cars in the sweltering heat.

It's time to work. It's time to commit to the processes and hustle. Enjoy it because one day you will look back and long for these difficult times.

The survival phase is all about taking your fledgling business and turning it into something that can support you and your family. We call it the survival phase because for many people, this is the phase when they go all in. In particular, if you go the side hustle route, this is when you give up your other job and focus solely on your cash practice.

This is the first phase when it becomes really important to get yourself organized. Sure, organization is important in general, but to go from 0–5K in revenue, you don't need much organization. This is also a phase when you have more time than you will once you hit phase 3. Take advantage of that time to set yourself up for success going forward.

By now you've figured some things out. You know how you like to interact with your patients. You have a basic understanding of how to sell yourself and how to get word-of-mouth referrals from your current patients. You've also probably got the hang of running workshops.

It's time to start documenting and organizing all of this. This is the time to start talking about standard operating procedures (SOP). If you're anything like me, you hear someone say SOP and you instantly want to fall asleep. Well, wake up. This shit is important even though you might not love it!

SOPs define how you want things to get done. You can have SOPs for lots of things. Here's a list of a few:

- How to structure your dress code
- How to do phone consults with potential patients
- How to ask for word-of-mouth referrals
- How to write the first patient email after an eval
- How the eval is structured
- How to organize your weekly schedule
- How to run workshops
- How to set up workshops
- How to follow up after workshops
- How to connect with local potential referral partners
- How to post a blog
- How to create a Facebook post
- How to put up an Instagram video
- What disposable materials you need and when they should be ordered

Your list will go on and on, but I think you get the point.

This is the time when you get to start defining these SOPs. The old approach would be to come up with an operations manual. You could do this and put it all in text form. I prefer to create videos. All you need is Zoom and Google Drive.

Use Zoom to record your screen and talk over either short presentations you put together or tasks you're doing on the computer. This was our approach, and it's allowed us to bring on PTs and easily train them in the basics of our booking/documenting system.

We've done this for tons of tasks and SOPs we have within our business. You should seriously consider taking this approach to your

SOPs at this state. The reality is, you have more than money right now. You have to use your time wisely. There are two areas you should focus your time on:

1. Developing relationships in your community to help with local referrals and lead generation. Become the go-to PT in your community for your specific niche; your business will thrive.

2. Defining your key tasks and the SOPs that you eventually want to teach to a PT you hire down the road.

Focus on these two areas and you'll be developing a solid foundation to build your practice on going forward.

In the next chapter, we'll go over an extremely pivotal phase. This is the phase when most people get stuck and have to make some hard decisions in order to continue growing.

CHAPTER 7

SUCCESS PHASE:
10–20K IN MONTHLY REVENUE

In the summer of 2015, my wife and I had a serious conversation about the direction we wanted to take with our business. We felt that we only had two options: Option 1 was to raise rates, stay small, and create a lifestyle business. Option 2 was to bring her into the business, expand, hire, and build a team.

This was a very difficult decision for us because we were in the success phase. We were regularly making 18–20K a month. We had low overhead, and we were in a really comfortable spot financially.

Let me take a second to define the difference between a lifestyle business and a true business.

A *lifestyle business* is a business that is started to get the business owner to a specific amount of income, and that's it. Basically, the business is designed to sustain your lifestyle. If you have very low cost of living, you could work only a few days a week and sustain your lifestyle. If you like really nice things and need to make more money, you can do this as well with a lifestyle business.

The demographic I see most commonly migrating to a lifestyle business is moms. Moms who want to be the primary caregiver of their kids have a really great opportunity with niche-based lifestyle businesses. My friend Carrie Pagliano in Washington, DC, is a perfect example of this. She has two to three days of patient-care hours only. These hours are based around her kids' schedule. This allows her the time she wants to spend with her kids yet still work as a PT. She also charges well over $200 an hour for client visits and is able to make more working part-time for herself than full-time for someone else. The lifestyle business is a pretty great deal if that's your intention with your business.

A *true business*, on the other hand, is a completely separate entity that functions when you're not around. This requires hiring staff, building a team, and managing significantly more resources to get developed. A true business is one that makes money when you're not there, and it's a true asset. By true asset, I mean something that someone else would be willing to buy one day.

I talk to a lot of business owners who think they have a true business but in actuality still have a lifestyle business. There's a litmus test for this. We call this the "hit by a bus" test, and it's pretty simple. If you were hit by a bus tomorrow, would your business still generate revenue, function, and continue to grow without you? If the answer is no, you have a lifestyle business. If the answer is yes, you have a true business.

Ashley and I made the difficult decision that we wanted to go for it and develop a true business. A business that would give us the opportunity to have both time and financial freedom. A business that, more importantly, would allow us the flexibility to spend more meaningful time with our kids than almost anyone else we know.

No matter what you decide to do, understand that a business is designed to allow you to live the life you want to live. You left an incredibly stressful job where you were seeing 25–30 people a day, writing notes for hours, and making decisions based on what some large insurance company told you you'd get reimbursed for.

The last thing you want to do is put yourself back into a stressful position that you hate. If you decide to make the decision to continue to grow a true business, understand there will be growing pains. It's just like when you were a kid. Your knees and shins started to ache, and it was really uncomfortable. All of a sudden you were 2 inches taller at the end of the summer and a hell of a lot better at basketball! Growing pains are necessary for fast changes both in our bodies and in our businesses.

We had some serious growing pains with Athletes' Potential. So much so that at the end of 2015, we almost went out of business.

In the summer of 2015, Ashley and I decided to go all in on our business and develop a true business. We wanted something that we could grow; and, in particular, we wanted employees. Not because we wanted someone to work for us but because we saw firsthand how many of my colleagues hit burnout and started to dislike their careers at PT by around three to five years out of school. We felt that we had developed a model to allow these PTs to both love what they do again and to bring them financial success at the same level as—or even a level above—their peers.

In order to grow into this new vision we had for Athletes' Potential, we needed to do a few things. First, we needed to expand into a larger space.

My office in a CrossFit gym had been totally fine for us to start the business. It wasn't the nicest space—most CrossFit gyms aren't—however, it was cheap and convenient. The biggest problem with the gym office was that we couldn't control our patient experience as well as we wanted to. We had no one greeting patients as they came in. We shared a common patient waiting area, and it was a bit confusing for new patients when they came in the building. We wanted to keep this office, but we also knew we needed our own standalone facility.

Searching for our first standalone space was both exciting and frustrating. It took us about three months to find the space that would work for us and a landlord willing to accept us. That might sound a bit odd, but the reality is, just because you want to sign a lease doesn't mean the landlord wants your type of business. We were actually turned down at three different spaces in the city before we finally got accepted into a space in the city of Decatur, Georgia. Decatur is in Eastside Atlanta, and our other office is in Westside Atlanta. We felt this would allow us to be more convenient to clients, so we pulled the trigger on the lease.

Mistake #1: We did not use a commercial realtor or a real estate attorney during this process. We felt we could do all of this on our own, and we lost out on thousands of dollars in concessions toward build out and free rent initially because of this. By the way, a commercial realtor costs you nothing. The fees for their services are paid by the landlord. This was a seriously dumb mistake I hope you learn from.

Right as we were in the process of getting the lease signed for the new space, we were also doing two other things. First, we were getting our plans drawn up for our build out of the space. Second, we were interviewing for our first full-time administrative position.

The build out process is another frustrating area where you can learn a lot of things the hard way. First of all, everyone tells you things will move faster than they actually do. We signed our lease October 1, 2015. We didn't officially open this new space until March 1, 2016. Yes, this is an incredibly long time, and it cost us a significant amount of money.

As for hiring our first full-time staff member, that also happened in October. We brought our first employee, Claire, on and … had no place for her to work. She worked remotely until March. We spent a significant amount of time training her on the tasks we wanted her to handle. We had her do as much work remotely as possible but, honestly, we lost a lot of money again by hiring her under the expectations that our build out would be done by December.

Mistake #2: Don't time hiring for a new facility until you at least get all the permitting done by the city you are building in. This basically means the city has approved your plans and the build out can begin. This is exactly what set us back so far. Once we got the plans approved, the build out phase didn't take very long at all—it was getting the permits that delayed the process. When dealing with your local government for anything, allow twice as much time as you initially think you need. That's how you create a realistic time frame.

Between our new overhead with the facility, equipment we had bought that was sitting unused, and a new full-time employee who had no place to work, we were hemorrhaging money. We took a huge step backward financially during this time to the tune of about $80,000.

I remember sitting on the couch with my wife one night in February of 2016. As you might imagine, we were both stressed. The past few months had been the most difficult and unhappy months of our marriage. The stress of a money-losing business doesn't just affect the business, it affects the entire family. We sat there looking at our business bank account and calculated just how many months we could keep this up before we had no cash left in the bank. We figured that we could make it through April 2016 on the cash reserves we had in the bank. After that we would have to start maxing out our credit cards or call it quits on Athletes' Potential. Neither of these were options we wanted to pursue.

Our build out was officially completed in February 2016, and we had one last step. We had to get our certificate of occupancy from the city, which took a couple more agonizing weeks. There's nothing worse than staring at a sparkling new facility full of equipment but not being able to use it. Until you get your certificate of occupancy, you are not allowed to use the facility for business. Finally, we got everything approved by the city, and we officially opened our Decatur office.

We needed that month of March 2016 to be a big month to help offset all the money we had lost in the expansion process. I remember that month very well. We had previously averaged around twenty new patients a month at our old office. After we opened our new office, we had forty new patients in the month of March. We had even raised our rates in conjunction with the new facility being open. We had our best month to that point and instantly offset much of the loss we had sustained with all of our build out mistakes.

Book recommendation #2: *The Obstacle Is the Way* by Ryan Holiday. If you've ever gone through an incredibly stressful time, this book will resonate with you. I'm a big believer in the fact that difficult events create opportunities for us to grow and improve. This book will be the perfect read as you're going through any challenging phase of business growth.

Friends who know what we went through at the end of 2015 ask me if I wish I hadn't decided to expand our business. My answer is and will always be that I wouldn't change what we did or how we did it. Yes, we made a lot of mistakes. Yes, we lost a lot of money. We also learned an incredible amount about what we didn't know.

From the start of our business, we had very little difficulty becoming successful. As nice as this sounds, it gave me a false sense of confidence that I knew what I was doing in business. This is a dangerous place to be. It's kind of like thinking you know how to swim because you crush it in a kiddie pool. Well, as soon as you jump in the deep end, things change. That's exactly what happened to me when I decided to expand.

CHAPTER 8

TURNING PRO AND BUILDING A TEAM PHASE: 20-40K IN MONTHLY REVENUE

Losing a significant amount of money and going through such a difficult expansion was a metaphorical business punch to the nuts. That phase made me realize some very important things. First, I was putting my company in danger by lacking business skills I desperately needed. Second, no matter how good of a PT I might have been, it would not help me grow our business past just myself. Third, I needed help, and I needed it right away.

This is the phase of my business journey in which I finally went out to find business mentorship. I did this through a number of different avenues. The easiest and cheapest way I found to improve my business knowledge was reading. I would read two business books a month and listen to another two business books on Audible every month.

The other way I worked on my business skill set was with an actual business coach. I found this coach through one of the books I read.

Book recommendation #3: *The E-Myth* by Michael Gerber. Definitely one of the top three books I recommend to anyone looking to get into entrepreneurship. Get it, read it, and apply it to your business.

During the spring of 2016, I applied to the EMyth Coaching Program. I didn't know much about business coaching but had played sports my entire life. The idea of being coached was familiar to me, and many of my business colleagues recommended I find a coach or mastermind group.

To say I had sticker shock when I talked to their sales rep on the phone is an understatement. I had no idea how much business coaching or mastermind groups typically cost, but I found out that day. To work with one of their coaches, it would cost me $1,500 a month and would require a one-year commitment. I didn't exactly have an extra $1,500 lying around in my business each month, but I did realize that I had a significant knowledge gap I needed to improve.

I pulled the trigger on the program and had about a week before the first onboarding call with my coach. I had some content that I needed to get through and had to send them a bunch of difficult things to define in my business. They wanted to know my deep internal reason for starting and growing my business. They wanted to know my three-, five-, and ten-year goals. They wanted to know exactly what I dreamed my life would look like going forward. They even asked me to write my own obituary. Seriously, writing a page-long obituary for myself might be one of the most uncomfortable things I've ever done.

Here's what they really did for me. They made me take a step back and realize that I needed to get good at *business*, not just physical therapy. It was time for me to turn pro and start building a team of people to take Athletes' Potential to the next level.

This phase is all about working on yourself and working on your business. In order for you to get to monthly revenue numbers of 20–40K in a 100% cash practice, you have to have a team. This is going to require solid admin staff and at least one more PT, depending on whether you are still seeing patients or not.

To build your team during this phase, you have to start with a strong administrative team. You may have hired your first administrative member in the previous phase. If so, that's great, but now it's time to make sure they are the right fit and helping facilitate the growth of your business.

These admin positions can seem like a cost to most people. They do cost money to have because you have to pay them a salary. But you also have to calculate the return on that investment. How many hours does a good admin free up for you? How many more patients can you work with? How many more high-level tasks can you complete? A good admin will more than pay for themselves.

The biggest mistakes I see during this phase are hiring mistakes. Too often people hire their friends or do little work to find the right fit. Business owners also assume that once they hire, it's the end of the process. They think if you just bring someone on and pay them, they'll fix all your problems. Well, that's not the reality of what happens. Once you hire someone, it's just the beginning of the work, and the process of training them never stops.

You have to have clear roles that you want this person to fill. They have to have structure but not be micromanaged. People are smart and will figure out solutions to the problems the business is facing, but they need to know what borders to function within. General George Patton famously said, "Never tell people how to do things. Tell them what to do and they will surprise you with their ingenuity."[2]

The most success we have had in terms of hiring has been based off our core values and personality. You can train skills, but you can't change someone's personality. This goes for both admin and PT staff. You want someone who exemplifies your core values. These are your deeply rooted core beliefs about what your company stands for. Having solid core values is one of the most important things you can do both for hiring and for showing people what you stand for.

This phase is all about building your core team. These people should be the nucleus of your company and bleed your core values. If you

---

2   "George S. Patton Quotes," BrainyQuote, https://www.brainyquote.com/quotes/george_s_patton_106027.

get this step right, your company will be in a great position to grow, scale, and continue to be successful in the future. Get this wrong and it can be twice as costly and time-consuming to fire and rehire these roles. Do not overlook the hiring process.

CHAPTER 9

REPEAT AND REFINE PHASE: 40K+ IN MONTHLY REVENUE

At the time I'm writing this book, this is the phase Athletes' Potential is currently in. We have four PTs and two admin team members. We use freelancers and consultants for things like graphic design, videography, digital marketing, and finance. Our team is lean, and that's the way we like it.

People think you need a million-dollar business to have financial and time freedom. That's just not true. Of course we expect to exceed seven figures in yearly revenue in the near future, but you don't need to do that to live a really great life. With good profit margins, this type of business can be a phenomenal thing to own. You get to have a huge impact on your community and have a simple, profitable business.

Here's the other really important thing that happens when you make it to this phase. You get ultimate say over what you do, when you do it, and how much of it you do.

My wife, Ashley, runs the administrative and operational side of our business. She can choose to work eight hours a day if she wants. She can also choose to go to the gym each day at ten in the morning to jump in the ladies class. She can leave whenever she wants if we need to get our kids or take them on a field trip. This allows both of us to be really involved in our kids' lives.

My schedule looks much different now as well. When I first started, I would see patients 30–35 hours a week and work on the business at night or before anyone woke up. I worked myself so much that I let my health suffer. I slept very little and sacrificed a lot to get our company going. Now I walk my son to school during the week. I prioritize time to train and stay healthy. I schedule ten patient visits per week, not because I have to but because I want to. When Ashley and I decide we want to take our kids on a trip, we do it. Our business still runs and is profitable even when we are not around. We spend more meaningful time with our kids than anyone else we know. We decide what we want to do or not do. This phase of business is all about having control and learning what you need to focus on.

This phase of business also has its own set of challenges, though. First, you have to switch your role from player to coach. No longer can you be the one doing all the work. You have to take a step back, figure out why you have been successful, and teach that to your staff. You have to learn to be a leader. That means there are probably some significant areas where you need to improve, or else they will create more problems for you.

Most of my time is spent working on how we can better run our business. How can we continue to grow our revenue so we can provide better benefits, salaries, and employment opportunities for our staff? I spend a lot of time testing, tracking, and making small changes to core processes. This could be as simple as tweaking how we answer a phone call or as complex as working on elaborate marketing campaigns with consultants.

All this time freedom has also allowed me to pursue other business ventures such as business consulting for physical therapists. This is work that I really get energized from, and I realize this is the area where I can have the biggest impact on our profession. Even having the time to write this book comes from the time freedom created with a properly structured true business. I guess I could stop working if I wanted to, but that sounds terrible. That sounds like a life with no meaning and no progression. I can't see that ever happening because

I really do enjoy this type of work. Regardless, it's up to you how you spend your time. In this phase of business, you just have to focus on how to take yourself out of the business. When you do that, you give yourself options.

My goal with this book is to help all of you realize that you can start a business and go out on your own. You can and should also focus on eventually taking yourself out of your business. You want to create that true business that allows you both time and financial freedom. The rest of this book covers two key areas you need to improve.

These areas are *marketing* and *sales*. If you don't have any new patients, you need this to fill your schedule. If you have a lot of new patients, you need this to get more and fill the schedules of your employees. Marketing and sales are the most important areas of focus in any business looking to thrive.

If your goal is to get to phase 5 of a performance-based cash practice, the next two sections will help you get there.

SECTION 2:

MARKETING

CHAPTER 10

DEFINING YOUR NICHE

The best marketing strategy ever ... care.
—Gary Vaynerchuk

Marketing in a nutshell is how you communicate why your prospective customers should come and work with you. It's how you get people through the door. You could be the world's greatest clinician and get everyone better. If no one knows who you are, you'll have an empty schedule.

I've met business owners in different niches and hear them brag about not even marketing their business. To them, this is a badge of honor. This is very common in CrossFit gyms. They view not marketing and solely relying on word of mouth as some kind of unheard-of feat. The reality is these business owners don't even know how to market, but their clients like their product/service so much that they generate word-of-mouth referrals.

Take that same business that gets great word-of-mouth referrals. If they added even some basic organization to their marketing, they could double their business in a matter of a year or two.

When I first started Athletes' Potential, I knew exactly the niche I wanted to work with. That niche was CrossFit, and about 90% of the people I saw my first year were CrossFitters. I did this because I felt I had a unique understanding of the sport as well as the skill set to help these athletes. Though it was unintentional, focusing on a specific niche was one of the smartest things I did when starting the practice. The more clearly you can define and inform potential patients on who you are the best choice for, the easier you make their buying decision.

When you go into a cash or out-of-network PT model, you cannot initially do so as a generalist. Let that soak in for a second. You might have gone through advanced training, have some cool letters behind your name, and think you can help pretty much anyone. That might be true, but you will be shooting yourself in the foot if you start a new practice with the intention of being the city's best generalist. You have to define a niche and dominate that niche; then you can make lateral transfers into general work or other niches.

Let's start by defining the niche you should focus on.

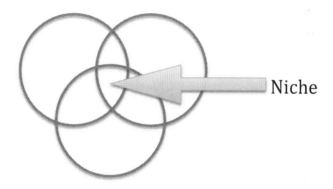

Niche

To define your niche, we'll go through a simple exercise. Look at the drawing above for a visual representation of this drill.

First, start by drawing three circles that intersect. Each of these three circles represents a part of your niche.

In Circle 1, write: I can help.
In Circle 2, write: I like them.
In Circle 3, write: Willing to pay.

Let's take my initial niche, CrossFit, as an example. For some of you, this might be the exact niche you decide to start with. When

I moved to Atlanta to open Athletes' Potential, I had been doing CrossFit myself for about five years. I had experience working with CrossFit competition teams, and I was one of the instructors for Kelly Starrett's MobilityWOD staff. This gave me a ton of unique knowledge and experience in this area. At the time, I also felt like this was an underserved niche with lots of CrossFit athletes just being told to stop doing CrossFit.

Here's what else I know about people who train CrossFit: First, they are borderline crazy about being able to train. When people say CrossFit is a cult, they are partially right. It's just a cult that harps on high-intensity exercise and will shame you if you walk into their gym with a bag of Chick-fil-A.

What's really unique about CrossFit is the group dynamic that develops. People get to know the other people working out with them pretty well. Misery loves company, and most CrossFit workouts are miserable. Because of this, people want to get back to that group and back to that training style as fast as possible. This is a good thing for someone who can help decrease pain and keep these athletes healthy. **So, for Circle 1: yes, I can help this niche.**

Over the past few years, I had spent a lot of time both training and coaching CrossFit. Some really good friends of mine I had met in CrossFit gyms. There's also a certain personality type that gravitates toward CrossFit, and I tend to like being around most of those people. Honestly, if you've trained CrossFit for a while, you can probably pick other CrossFitters out in airports. They're the people wearing Lululemon shorts and T-shirts and walking around in Reebok Nanos. They might be doing air squats in the corner while they wait for their flight to board or doing some couch stretch work at an empty terminal gate. These are people I like to be around, and I like working with them. **So, for Circle 2: yes, I enjoy being around these people.**

Lastly, CrossFit isn't cheap. Most gyms cost between $120 and $250 a month. CrossFitters also have no problem buying a $50 jump rope, $200 pair of Olympic lifting shoes, $100 worth of bright-blue knee sleeves, and $80 a month worth of only the finest grass-fed whey protein. My point is, they pay for all kinds of shit because they love CrossFit and want to get better at CrossFit. I know this niche has a certain amount of disposable income available just to be part of a CrossFit gym. That means they have money to pay me when they hurt their back deadlifting. **So, Circle 3: yes, they can pay to work with me.**

Go through this drill on your own, and think of a few different niches that might fit this criteria. In particular, if you have a special skill in coaching or as an athlete, that can be very helpful. Let's imagine you were a collegiate runner. You may have a very unique viewpoint and significant credibility with the running community. Let's say you also like to work with golfers. If this sounds like you, don't try and make your name working with golfers at first. Take the low-hanging fruit; you'll get connected with runners who want to work with you. Once you and your business gain a solid local reputation, you can make a lateral transfer to trying to get more golfers in. Building credibility in one niche makes it so much easier to expand to other niches in your area.

Before you try any slick marketing, make sure you know which niche you want to work with. If your brand messaging is clear, your marketing will be more effective. If your messaging is generalized, you will confuse people. It's totally fine to deter certain people by focusing on the people you really like, people you can help, and people who can pay for your services. This will allow only the most qualified people to actually talk to you or get to see you. This is exactly what you want, so make sure to define your niche first.

CHAPTER 11

DEFINING YOUR PERFECT CLIENT

Now that you know what niche you want to focus on, it's time to get granular on who your perfect client is. When I lived in Hawaii, I went sport fishing for my birthday one year. We wanted to catch a marlin, so when we considered the boat we wanted to charter, we looked specifically at boats that fished for marlin. There are plenty of charter boats in Hawaii. Many of them cater to different types of clientele. Some were for fun family outings, and some were for sport fishing. A few focused specifically on marlin, and those were the ones we checked out.

You want to be that marlin-specialized boat for your potential clients. If you're really clear on who you are the best at working with, you'll attract more of them and repel the others. That marlin sport fishing boat didn't want a family of four coming on board thinking they were going to catch some little snappers. They were for people looking to do one thing: catch a marlin. And they charged a premium for it.

This same approach can be used with our potential clients. Now that you have a defined niche, you can drill down even more and start to detail exactly who your potential target customer is.

To do this, we have our business consulting clients go through a perfect client avatar exercise. Get a piece of paper or a whiteboard and write out these characteristics:

- Age
- Gender
- Marital Status
- Occupation

- Income Level
- Kids Y/N
- Hobbies/Interests
- Values
- Dislikes
- Pain Points
- Fears and Worries

My perfect client avatar has changed over the years. It started with a much younger CrossFit athlete population and has evolved alongside our practice. The other thing that's important in this exercise is to give a name to this perfect client. The whole point of naming them and writing out all this detail is to be able to use it in your marketing efforts. Every time you write a blog post, you'll write it with your perfect client in mind. Whenever you do a video, it's for your perfect client. Whenever you put together a workshop, you should organize it in a way that would appeal to and help your perfect client.

Our perfect client is named Greg. He's a forty-eight-year-old attorney. He's married and has two kids. He makes over $200,000 a year. He was an athlete growing up and still wants to use his body in an athletic way to this day. He's interested in CrossFit, football, soccer, and golf, and he watches SportsCenter daily. He's got some previous injuries from his time playing sports and hates to avoid activities. He knows he's getting older but loves to keep up with his two high school–age daughters who both play soccer. When he gets together with his friends, he notices they're becoming less functional and more unhealthy. He loves his friends, but he doesn't want to go down the health path they've chosen. He wants to be active and be able to enjoy the financial success he's worked so hard for. He wants nothing to do with medication, surgery, or any other medical procedure he can avoid in the future.

Greg is our ideal customer, and when we market anything, it's to Greg. The funny thing is, if you do a good job of this, you'll end up with a bunch of people in your office that are similar to Greg—or whoever your ideal customer happens to be. That is actually a great barometer of how well you've defined your customer and marketed to them. If you have a bunch of twenty-six-year-old runners coming in to see you, but your ideal customer is Greg, something is off.

This is also a difficult exercise to do when you first get started. It may be helpful for you to redo this every six months in the early days of your business. It is also really helpful to have a client you love working with that you can use as a reference for this exercise. Just think of your favorite past patient. Think of the person you wish you had on your schedule every day. That's the person you want to define, and that's the person you want your marketing to attract.

CHAPTER 12

WHERE ARE THEY, AND HOW DO YOU REACH MORE OF THEM?

Now that you've defined your niche and your perfect customer, it's time to figure out where they are and how to get them in your office. This is what marketing companies charge a lot of money to do for you. Anyone or any company that can generate quality leads for a business is worth A LOT of money.

Marketing is an art and a science. It's very important that you track if what you're doing is working. Not tracking your marketing efforts is kind of like playing darts with your eyes closed. Every once in a while you might hit a bull's-eye, but you're not going to do it with much regularity.

I've had my fair share of bad experiences with marketing companies. I've gone through two marketing companies that I thought would be the solution I was looking for. That solution was more new patients than we could handle.

Company #1 was a traditional digital marketing firm that focused mostly on Search Engine Optimization (SEO). They set up specific landing pages and primarily used paid Google ads to drive traffic to our site and the landing pages they created. They told us they could get our phone ringing off the hook. Well, they were right about that; our phone did ring like crazy. The problem was, it was primarily spam and leads that were a terrible fit for our company. We stuck with it for about six months and had basically nothing positive to show for it. Frustrated and disappointed with the outcome, we moved on to company #2.

Company #2 was what would be considered a content marketing company. They primarily focused on blogs, videos, and social media. We had been doing a ton of this from day one, so we seemed like a perfect fit for them. All the hard work was already done since at the time we had well over 100 blogs and over 200 videos on YouTube and Facebook. We also had an active email list of previous customers. I very much preferred this company's approach, and I was more involved in their process than I was with the first company. They helped us out a lot with better organization of our email list, generating leads via contact forms, and adding structure to our content creation.

The only problem with this company was they would only work with us if we started implementing a software platform called Infusionsoft. This is an incredibly powerful platform, but no one on our staff was able to get the hang of it very well. That meant that all the Infusion-soft tasks needed to be done by this marketing company. Even simple things like putting together a weekly newsletter had to go through this company. These extra costs added up quickly. We also constantly needed to go back and adjust our marketing verbiage. This happened primarily because they had no clinical experience and really didn't understand what we did in our office.

The nail in the coffin for us was when our account manager left. We really liked her more than the owner of the company. When she left, we decided to take our marketing in-house. This has been my primary role in our company ever since. I'm a strong believer that marketing is a skill all business owners need to work on. It is the driver of new business to your practice. You may work with a team to implement your approach, but you have to have the vision of what they are working on. You cannot leave this up to others to figure out for you. Become obsessed with marketing and your business will thrive.

At the time of writing this book, Athletes' Potential has had approximately 500 new patients in the past twelve months. That puts us at an average of about forty new patients per month. This is while being in network with no insurance companies and being a 100% cash pay clinic.

So, the million-dollar question is: How the hell do you get forty new cash-paying clients per month?

To do this, we use a three-part marketing approach shown in the pyramid below. We'll define the elements of this pyramid in detail in the next few chapters.

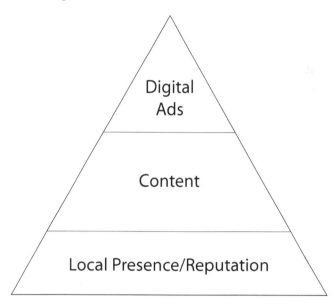

CHAPTER 13

BUILDING YOUR DREAM TEAM

I hate networking. If you put me in a room with fifty people I don't know, I'm a totally different person. I seriously turn into an idiot who has no social skills. I'm also very comfortable by myself. I don't need to have people around me to feel happy. In fact, I crave isolation in certain circumstances. Much of this is probably due to the number of times I moved as a kid. When you go to nine different schools before you graduate high school, you get used to being by yourself.

Now, if you put me in a setting with a couple people who all have common interests, I'm in my natural element. I really enjoy getting to go deep, learning about other people in a less-crowded setting. I prefer to have fewer relationships but to have those relationships be very meaningful.

This is an important thing to know about yourself; take a step back to see what type of environment you function best in. You might love meeting new people. You might get a ton of energy from attending networking events and connecting with all kinds of different professionals. If that's your personality type, you would thrive in a setting like a chamber of commerce meeting or city business group networking events.

If you're more like me, you'll thrive in small group settings. This is where things like local masterminds, small entrepreneur groups, and one-on-one meetings are a much better fit for me. Either way, you have to get out of your office and meet people in your community.

One thing to keep in mind is that not all relationships are equal. Some will be much more impactful on your business than others. In my experience, getting to know fifty local professionals and business owners at a networking event is not as important as having a strong relationship with one complementary business owner.

I call this "Assembling your Dream Team."

When I think about a Dream Team, I think back to when I played sports growing up. The Dream Team was a famous U.S. Olympic basketball team that dominated in the nineties. I realize writing this that I feel old because many of you reading this probably were born after the Dream Team's time.

Like the Dream Team, the best teams I've been part of had good players that worked well together. There was also some overlap in skills of different players on the team. A point guard and a shooting guard on a basketball team function in different positions. That being said, they both need to be able to dribble, pass, and shoot the ball. Their roles are slightly different, but they complement each other.

In this scenario, building your Dream Team means building your network of complementary service providers. When I looked at assembling my Dream Team in Atlanta, it was solely for the purpose of having a network of the absolute best people I could refer my clients to. I once heard Gray Cook say: "You get 100% of the blame for a bad referral and 50% of the credit for a good one." That is absolutely true, and it's the reason I have been so particular about who we've added to our team.

Your team doesn't have to be big. It can be as small as five to ten people. Traditionally, PTs have tried to form relationships with physicians so they can cultivate referral relationships. These are not the types of relationships I'm referring to when I talk about building your Dream Team. These are selfless relationships that you're forming for the purpose of getting a better outcome for your patients.

Here's a list of some professionals you can aim to have on your Dream Team:

- Ortho doctors
- Family practice doctors
- Functional medicine providers
- Non-surgical sports medicine doctors
- Other PTs that have complementary skill sets
- Chiropractors
- Massage therapists
- Sports psychologists
- Dietitians
- Trainers
- Coaches
- Fitness facility owners

You may have already started building your Dream Team, or you may just be getting started. Maybe you don't know anyone yet. Whatever the case, I want you to do this exercise. Reach out to people you do know, and ask if they have any recommendations for people that fit these subcategories. Also, do your own research. See what kind of content those people have put out. Look at their website and social proof. Look at these professionals as if you were a client who was considering making an appointment.

Once you have your potential Dream Team list mapped out, it's time to start making contact with these people. You can do this via email, phone call, or even social media. It doesn't matter how you do it, but understand there's a strong likelihood you'll get turned down at first. Most of these really high-quality people are busy. You have to lead with value in a way that helps them to start developing the relationship.

For a gym owner or trainer in your area, this could mean offering comped visits to learn about their approach with their clients.

With a doc, this could be setting up a time to learn about what types of patients they are the best at working with. You could even talk to their office manager or key staff member; it doesn't have to be the actual doc. In many cases, they will be the hardest to connect with.

If you really want to get in front of someone, make an appointment. I've done this with multiple massage therapists, docs, and trainers when I was trying to meet people I thought would be good members of my Dream Team. This works really well. First, you're showing that you value their time. You're also showing that you value their skills. It might cost you some money, but it's a great way to lay a foundation for a future relationship.

Once you make contact and get some face time, don't screw it up. Here's what I mean by that: People are inherently selfish. We all like to talk about ourselves and get things from other people. It's human nature, and you need to check that at the door before you meet with someone you want on your Dream Team. You have to lead with adding something to their business or helping them become more successful.

This could mean helping promote something they are doing. This could mean referring the right people their way without asking for something in return. This could mean sending them relevant information about a topic they expressed interest in.

Let me give you an example featuring a massage therapist who is on our Dream Team. I had been told by multiple people that this guy was great. He was also crazy busy, so I booked a session with him. I figured I could use it, and it would give me a chance to see firsthand how he works with people. Turns out he was great, and

I found out we shared similar continuing education interests. He was a big fan of my mentor, Kelly Starrett. At the time, Kelly's new book *Deskbound* was about to be published. This massage therapist expressed interest in getting the new book when it came out. I had actually been sent two copies of *Deskbound* before it was released since I teach for Kelly's group. The next day, I brought him over one of the advance copies I had and gave it to him. I asked for nothing in return. I never mentioned him referring patients to us, and to this day I've never asked him to send someone our way.

That one relationship has helped us tremendously, both in reputation and in patient volume. I send people his way who are looking for a fairly aggressive massage therapist who works with athletes. He sends people our way who want dry needling and need advanced corrective movement work. We send people to him not because he sends people our way; we send people to him because he's the best at what he does in our area.

Another example would be the functional medicine doc on our Dream Team. She has been a huge asset to our company and has helped solve some very difficult problems.

About three years ago, I read a book called *Brain Maker*, which is all about the gut-brain connection. This book changed the way I looked at functional or integrative medicine. It also changed the way I looked at chronic pain, and I started delving much more into food/gut issues with chronic pain patients. I started noticing a strong correlation between gut issues and chronic pain. I didn't have the desire or time to learn everything I could about functional medicine. I did realize it was important, though, and I knew we needed to add a specialist in that area to our Dream Team.

I reached out to a prior patient of mine who was a dietician. I asked her if she knew any good functional med docs, and she said yes.

She recommended a group that was a few miles north of our office. When I reached out to them about meeting with the main physician, I was denied. I tried to explain to them that I had a pretty busy cash practice and I was interested in potentially sending some of our clients to their clinic. The office manager was tough, and she still denied me. She did offer me a consolation prize: she set me up with one of the nurse practitioners who worked there.

I worked with tons of amazing nurse practitioners when I was in the Army, so I jumped at the chance to meet this provider. When we met, I knew this person was the perfect fit for our Dream Team. She had gone to the same undergrad college as me, she had previously worked as a personal trainer like I had, and she was incredibly smart. We immediately started sending people to their clinic and always recommended they see this nurse practitioner in particular.

Eventually, this provider left that group and started her own practice. We still send people her way and always get a great response from our patients that work with her. Again, I've never once asked her to send people my way. It's not about that. It's about the fact that we think she is the best fit for our population. She makes us look good, and her business grows because of it. We definitely see people referred by her, but we'd honestly send people her way no matter what. This is the approach you need to take with these relationships.

Your Dream Team is about building a group of the best complementary professionals you can find. The more you focus on serving your clients and the less you focus on getting referrals, the faster you will start building long-lasting relationships.

The action item from this chapter is to start right now. Start finding these Dream Team members, and start building your relationships. The Internet could go away tomorrow, and Facebook could just decide to shut down all of a sudden. If you have a solid Dream Team in place, the digital changes won't affect your business. Your business will be more secure, and you'll get the best possible outcomes for you clients.

Start building your Dream Team today!

CHAPTER 14

LOCAL PRESENCE AND REPUTATION

In the past few years I've had an opportunity to consult with hundreds of clinicians looking to start, grow, and run their own cash practice. One common theme I've recognized in all of those conversations is that a local presence can make or break your business.

There are two PTs that I started working with a little over a year ago. They have the same clinical skills, a very similar personality, and they started their practices around the same time.

PT #1 starts his practice in an office in a gym on the West Coast. He coaches at the local gym, does local events/workshops, and networks with his local community. A year into starting his practice, he's averaging about 8K in revenue per month.

PT #2 starts his practice in an office in a gym on the East Coast. He coaches at the local gym, does local events/workshops, and networks with his local community. A year into starting his practice, he's averaging about 15K in revenue per month.

Both of these PTs charge the same per visit and have similar demographics in their cities. So, what's the big difference between the two? PT #1 is from the Midwest and moved to the West Coast to start his practice. PT #2 was born and raised in the city where he started his practice.

You cannot underestimate the value of deep relationships in a local business. It can seriously make or break your practice. You are at a significant advantage if you are from an area and very well connected there. This is not just true for a physical therapy practice but for any type of business you open. You could open a mediocre restaurant, but if people know you and really like you, they will support it because they want to support you.

Now, I'm not telling you that you can only open a PT practice in your hometown. I don't even have a hometown. My dad was in the Army, and we moved every few years. What I'm telling you is that the number and depth of local relationships you have will directly affect the success of your business.

If there is one mistake I see over and over again with PTs that fail in private practice, it's that they do not prioritize their local relationships. Too often they think that if they open an office, people will come. This is a dangerous strategy and can lead to the failure of your business.

The other mistake I see is PTs thinking they can rely on paid ads (Google and Facebook) to grow their business and get new patients. This just doesn't work, and here's why.

You really wanted some pizza. You're on Facebook scrolling through your news feed, and all of a sudden you see a sponsored post for a pizza place. Now, do you just click the button and buy some pizza? If you're like most consumers, that's not what you do.

First, you click their post and check out their Facebook page. They only have 100 likes on their page, so you instantly have less interest in this potential pizza purchase. Next you go to Yelp and look up this restaurant. There's only one review, and it seems too positive, so you assume the owner probably wrote it himself. In a last-ditch effort, you text your friend who also loves pizza and ask if he's ever heard of the place; he says no. So you decide to just call the pizza place you always order from, and that new pizza place loses a potential repeat customer.

This scenario is what happens inside the mind of real human

beings. We are tricky, fickle people to deal with, especially on digital platforms. We are so used to being sold to online now, we just assume everyone is trying to scam us.

Now, let's take this same scenario and imagine that, instead of 100 likes on their Facebook page, this new pizza place had 1,000 likes. When you went to Yelp, they had fifteen really compelling reviews. Lastly, you called your buddy who loves pizza, and he tells you that place is amazing and you totally need to try it. The outcome of this scenario would turn into a successful digital ad for that pizza place.

I can tell you this much: selling pizza is a shitload easier than selling physical therapy, especially cash physical therapy. If you do not have a strong local presence, all of your other marketing efforts will be less effective.

Because of this, we spend a significant amount of time and resources on local relationship development. I am not originally from Atlanta. I moved here specifically because I wanted to open a practice and they had an airport that was really easy to get direct flights out of. All of the relationships we have are a result of time, effort, and consistency. Below is an example of how to build your local presence and gain a rock-solid reputation in your community.

Early on, CrossFit is what I spent most of my time working on. When I moved to Atlanta, I printed out a map of all the CrossFit affiliates in the city. I then recorded the name/contact info of all the gym owners from their website. I asked the gym owner where I was leasing space if he knew any of the people on the list I created. He actually knew quite a few of them, and I asked him if he could make a warm introduction to a few of them via email.

I got him to introduce me through email to about five gym owners. I reached out to them and only heard back from about three of those gym owners. I positioned myself as the CrossFit injury expert in the city of Atlanta and set up a time to meet with them. This meeting was for me to get a better idea of how they ran their gym and their programming, and to learn who their ideal customer was. I told them I was going to be working with a lot of people that were injured but looking to get back into a gym. I wanted to make sure to send these people to the right gym.

You have to lead with value, and I led with wanting to see if they would be good gyms to refer people to. This means, I would potentially be sending them business. This is what frequently happens with our patients; they're injured and frustrated. We get them pain-free, and then they want to get in better shape. That means they need to go to a gym, and they very much trust our opinion on which gym to go to.

Now, when I met with these first couple gym owners, I set it up so we could talk after a workout. I actually took one of their classes, saw how the coach worked, and then talked to them afterward about a few things.

First, I just wanted to get a better idea of their background. How did they get into this business, and what were their goals. I made 90% of the conversation about them and what type of client was ideal for their gym. I really hit it off with two of the three original gym owners I met with. The third I could tell was not the right fit for me, and it was not a place I would feel comfortable referring people.

With these two, I offered to further the relationship with more value. I offered them a few sessions for free with me so they could get a better idea of my approach. They both had little things they were dealing with and were happy to take me up on the offer.

Over the next few weeks, I saw both of these gym owners and was able to move the relationship one step further. As they started to see results with the techniques I was teaching them, I mentioned that I teach local workshops. They were both really excited about hosting a workshop at their gym. I set these up and was able to get new patients from each of the workshops I taught at these facilities.

Once I got to the point where they knew I was able to help their clients and they had a good experience with a workshop, I asked them for some help. I asked them if they knew any other trainers or gym owners in the city they thought I should meet with. They both had recommendations and again made warm introduction between these people and me.

I repeated this whole process again and again for years. Many of these introductions and relationships were busts. People either wanted nothing to do with me, or they were not the right fit for our client base. Either way, I have had plenty of non-productive meetings over the past few years. You cannot expect everyone to like you or want to have anything to do with you from a business standpoint. The people who succeed are those who can take rejection better than others.

I would take ten meetings if I knew I would end up with one beneficial long-term relationship. Some of the original people I met years ago are still people I consider friends today. This is so important. *You have to develop friendships with other business owners.* Your friends want to see you succeed. Your friends will go out of their way to help you. Your friends will stick up for you if someone has something bad to say about your business. The more friends you have in a local business, the more success you will have.

We currently focus on our local presence and reputation in a few different ways. First, we still connect regularly with people we've worked with for years. This could be coaches, trainers, barbers, local business owners, and other professionals. Next, we still teach local workshops all over the city. We typically put on two to four workshops every month. This has gotten much easier now that we have four PTs. Lastly, we still take part in our local community activities by practicing what we preach. We run local races, train at local gyms, buy equipment from local vendors, and attend local networking events. We can't go to a local festival without running into a half dozen old patients, and it's amazing. We are genuinely part of the local community, and you can't fake that.

Your local presence is something that's time intensive and can be scary to work on at first. There is a reason why this is the base of our marketing pyramid. Even without content or digital ads, we would still get 20+ new patients a month just from word-of-mouth referrals and recommendations from local relationships. Before you go getting into the world of paid ads, you'd better make sure you have this part of the pyramid in place.

CHAPTER 15

WORKSHOPS

All the great speakers were bad at first.
—Ralph Waldo Emerson

When I moved to Atlanta to open Athletes' Potential, I pretty much knew no one. My wife has some family living here, but they had no involvement in healthcare or the niche I was focusing on. I grossly underestimated how much work it would take to build my reputation in the city.

Before I transitioned from the Army into private practice, I had started working as an instructor for the MobilityWOD group. I had been teaching for about six months at that time, and one of our other instructors was Theresa Larson. Theresa and her husband, Per, own a successful cash practice called Movement Rx in San Diego. One piece of advice she gave me was to start teaching workshops at gyms. She recommended teaching the MWOD style approach to gym members for common injuries. Theresa was dead on with this recommendation, and I credit her advice with how we built our reputation in Atlanta.

So what do you do when you know very few people in a new city and you're trying to build a reputation? My solution was to teach a crazy amount of workshops, basically anywhere someone would have me. By crazy amount, I mean at least one workshop a week for the first six months I was in business. I taught over forty workshops in the span of six months. I did this mostly at CrossFit gyms, but I also taught at personal training studios, running stores, and local businesses. I would drive as far as an hour away just to teach a workshop. Here's the power of this.

With no other marketing plan in place, just doing workshops took me from zero to eighty patient visits per month by the time we were six months into the business. I had gone from $0 to well over $10,000 in monthly revenue by that sixth month. Workshops are a great lead generation option. We still to this day do at least two workshops a month. Here's why they work so well.

We live in a digital world. Everyone walks around with a computer in their pocket, is ultra-connected via social media, and has access to more information than someone can consume in a lifetime. One thing that hasn't changed is that we're all still humans, and human interaction is memorable.

Think of the last concert, football game, or comedy show you went to. Sure, you can watch these things on TV or listen to these bands on any number of streaming devices. The difference is the experience. No one has ever said, "Hey, remember when we were sitting in the car and that Dave Matthews Band song came on Spotify." But I'm sure plenty of people can vividly remember a live concert they went to, a time they watched their favorite band play.

The difference is the *live experience*. This difference is the same for in-person events versus digital content. The power of live events and experiences is what makes workshops convert so well; they are worth your time.

We use a three-part approach to workshops.

1. Setting them up.
2. Teaching the event.
3. Following up after the event.

I'll explain each in detail so you can follow our three-part approach to running a successful workshop.

Part 1: Setting up Workshops

Sometimes the hardest part of setting up workshops is getting people to say yes to hosting. This is a problem I ran into when I first started putting on workshops in Atlanta. Very few people knew who I was or what kind of information I could teach. They didn't know how I could be beneficial to their gym, and I got turned down a lot.

Here's the honest truth: You need to get used to being turned down. You need to get used to people not wanting to work with you. You need to accept the fact that some people aren't going to like you. This was very difficult for me when I started Athletes' Potential, and I still struggle with this today.

Everyone wants people to like them. If people say they don't care what others think, they're full of shit. It's the ability to deal with rejection that really matters. The only way to get used to being turned down is to get turned down often.

Here's the approach that has worked the best for me when it comes to getting workshops set up.

First, try and get warm introductions to potential workshop sites. These can be gyms, training studios, yoga studios, Pilates studios, government offices, and local businesses. You don't necessarily have to talk to the owner. Get in touch with a coach, trainer, admin personnel, or even someone who is a member of the facility you're trying to build a relationship with. You can teach workshops at any number of different locations. These warm introductions are key.

By warm introduction, I mean get someone you know to introduce you to someone else. This could be via email, phone, text, or in person. Early on, this may mean asking friends and family or current clients if they know anyone who fits what you're looking for. It's all about getting those first couple locations; it will snowball from there.

You'd be surprised how powerful your network is. The problem is, no one ever uses it. They just sit in their office by themselves and hope people will come; they never *ask for help*. Plenty of people will want to help you—you just have to ask them.

Once you've gotten an intro to a potential workshop host, it's time to meet them. Don't go in and ask right away to run a workshop in their facility. This is just like marketing. You're trying to move people from cold to warm and, eventually, to hot. Rushing this can ruin the relationship.

This is where your ability to communicate with others will come in handy. Some people may be very interested in doing a workshop with you from day one. These are the *hot leads*. Most will not be like this, and you'll need to further the relationship. The best way we've found to do this is to work with that lead one-on-one to show them your skills. This is about the only time I'll ever give something away for free. Comping a potential key relationship a few visits can have a huge return on investment in the long run.

The other great way to further the relationship is to show a willingness to learn and train. Think of a CrossFit gym. If you show up at a CrossFit gym and talk to the owner about running a workshop to stop people from getting hurt, they'll probably want nothing to do with you. If you show up at that gym, train with them, and talk to the owner about how you can help improve movements with a workshop, they'll be a lot more likely to say yes. Sometimes you've gotta walk the walk to get them to say yes.

Once you've got some established relationships, you can then use those to leverage other potential workshop locations. Let's say you've just run a great workshop at a CrossFit gym. Afterward, make sure to ask the point of contact for that workshop if they know anyone else who they think would benefit from this workshop. This will eventually turn into a growing group of highly qualified contacts that can provide you with a location to teach multiple workshops.

The second important part of setting up workshops is getting people to show up. Having ten to thirty people in a gym ready to go through a workshop is a fun experience. If the energy level is high and people are interested in what you're saying, it's amazing. There's nothing worse than showing up to run a workshop for one person. This has happened to me—but it's not necessarily a total bust. That one person may end up being an amazing client of yours for years to come.

There are a few different ways to help improve the show-up rate of your workshop.

First, communicate with the workshop point of contact (probably the gym owner or coach) on what you're talking about. This will give them a really clear idea of how to present it to their members, explaining why they might want to come. You can also put together a one-page flyer explaining the workshop and send it to this person. They can put the flyer up in their gym or email it out to their list. They can also use this one-pager as a Facebook post. Most gyms have their own private Facebook groups. These can be really interactive and a great place to have the workshop host put out information.

Almost all of the workshops we run are closed. That means they are for the facility and its members only. This makes it very difficult to market if you can't get the host to help. You want to make sure the host understands this and you help them as much as possible.

Adding a small charge for the workshop is a strategy we have found to be very successful—it has helped us get as many as forty-five people to a workshop at a time. Usually this is $10 per person, but it could be whatever amount you want. Here's why this is effective:

1. It weeds out people that are absolutely the wrong fit for our

style of practice. If they aren't willing to spend $10 on a workshop, they'll definitely not be willing to spend $200 for a visit.

2. It creates a sense of inherent value. Not only do people have more perceived value to what you're teaching, but they'll also pay attention. They have some skin in the game at this point.

3. We let the host keep whatever revenue the workshop generates. This is one of the huge reasons hosts will market to their members. If they get twenty-five people to show up, they make an extra $250 that month. We teach an awesome workshop their members rave about, and they make a little extra money that month.

You can also host workshops at your own facility if you have one. This can be a great way to get people exposed to your location and your staff. These become a little more difficult to get people to. The marketing efforts fall on your shoulders. Because of this, we prefer to do workshops at other locations. It allows us to get more people to show up and expose our brand to new parts of the city.

We also love the opportunity to help generate some extra income for our partner gyms. If we can use our skill set to teach something impactful and they can make some money in the process, we will develop a really strong relationship. They'll have us back to do more workshops and tell more people about our business.

The central component of running a local service that businesses like is having strong relationships. If you're like me and aren't from the area where you run your business, this can be difficult. Workshops are a great way to get in front of the right people and cultivate solid relationships with complementary businesses in your area. If I could only pick one marketing tool to start my business over again, it would be workshops.

Part 2: Teaching the Workshop

In your marketing, you need to educate, entertain and execute.

—Billy Gene Shaw

So, you've networked, you got warm intros, and you've got a workshop or two set up. Now comes the fun part; you get to actually teach it. Remember these three things: educate, entertain, and execute.

The best presenter I've ever seen is Kelly Starrett. He's not a presenter in the traditional style like a Steve Jobs. His style is more raw and in-your-face. I've never seen him use a PowerPoint presentation or any sort of visual aid on a screen. Give the man an empty gym, a whiteboard, and two days. He'll change the way people see the world around them in regard to movement, rehab, and strength/conditioning.

I've had a chance to watch him teach a lot. To start working with the MobilityWOD team as an instructor, I had to attend half a dozen courses as an assistant. The content was roughly the same, but the way he presented it changed based on the area and population he was teaching. I took notes not only on the content I needed to memorize but also observed some of the subtle things Kelly did that made him such a dynamic speaker.

Between the hundreds of hours I've spent with Kelly and the hundreds of hours I've spent as an instructor myself, I've taken away a few key points to being a dynamic speaker. Implement these and you'll run effective, fun, and memorable workshops that draw new patients and grow your business.

Key #1: You have to entertain people, but you're not a stand-up comedian.

We all know people who are just funny. They are quick-witted and always seem to know the right thing to say. We also know people who think they are funny and constantly tell jokes or try to make others laugh. Which person should you be more like when you present?

When you present, you want to make sure you are memorable. But the way to be memorable is not to use silly, unrelated humor. An easy place to start is to compare different types of people. I always love to show the example of a hypermobile person versus a hypomobile person. It's funny and memorable for people to visually see the difference between these two types. Ask those same people to do a task that requires a decent amount of mobility and it becomes even more memorable.

Take, for instance, squatting with your feet together. This is something we believe people should be able to do, but you'd be surprised how few people can actually do it. If you teach a squat clinic or a foot/ankle clinic, compare two people squatting with their feet together. If you have one person with flexible ankles and one with tight ankles, the difference will be dramatic. People will laugh, but they will remember that you showed them how the limited range of motion affects a position that makes sense to them. They will remember this. They won't remember you trying to tell a joke and screwing up the punch line.

Key #2: No one knows more about what you're presenting than you.

The cool thing about teaching workshops you develop is that you'll know the material better than anyone there. When I was in my last year at Baylor, I had to defend the research we did while I was in school. This was an intimidating task, in particular because I was given the role of answering all the statistics questions. I barely passed statistics, and I'm not the best with math in general. I voiced this concern to our research director, and I'll never forget what he told me. He said, "Danny, you've been working on this for two years. There will literally be no one in the audience that knows more about this research than you." That gave me a ton of confidence, and I got through the research defense unscathed.

When you teach workshops or give any presentation, keep this in mind. The more confident you can be about your understanding of the material, the easier it will be for you to teach it. It's all about mindset. A confident mindset leads to a successful workshop.

Key #3: Command the room.

This can be a tough one for people, but it can make a huge difference. One thing I noticed when Kelly taught was that he always commanded the room's attention. When he spoke, he would pause and make eye contact. I remember the first course I went to, he did this to me. We were teaching at the Rogue Fitness Headquarters in Columbus, Ohio. He was giving the intro lecture for the Movement and Mobility Course he used to teach. Toward the end he paused and looked right at me. It felt like he looked at me and paused for ten seconds. It was probably only two seconds, but my heart started racing. In those two seconds, I didn't know if he was going to ask me a question, tell me I was doing something wrong, or tell me I had a stain on my shirt. After the pause and eye contact, he moved on to finish his point.

That moment showed me the power of two key principles to commanding a room.

First, you want to be confident. Don't fake confidence, but project real confidence; know exactly what you're going to teach, and people are going to love it. The way you walk, interact with others, and set up for a workshop shows it. People have an innate ability to read body language. We can tell when we see the body language of a confident person versus a non-confident person. You have to be confident to command a room.

Second, you have to force yourself to pause and make direct eye contact with people. I learned this at Rogue Fitness with Kelly, and he even told me how important this was over that weekend. He said he intentionally looked at me and paused during the intro. We talked about the power of that and how it made me feel. It was like someone giving me the cheat codes to public speaking success. When you're emphasizing an important point, make sure to pause longer than you think is necessary and make direct eye contact with people.

Key #4: Tell stories.

People love stories. It's something universal; people of all ages, from kids all the way to adults, love a good story. We also remember stories much better than we remember anything else. Just think of the story I told you about Kelly and me teaching in Columbus. I could have told you some statistic about improvement in audience engagement when you make eye contact, and you probably wouldn't remember it. You'll be much more likely to remember pausing and making eye contact when you think about Kelly staring me down from across the room.

People at workshops love stories; they respond really well to that approach. This works even better if you can align a relevant story with the topic and audience. This may be something that you'll have to spend time thinking about before the workshop, but it makes a huge difference.

Let's say I teach a lower back pain workshop at a local gym. I can talk about the mechanics of why back pain happens and teach some cool mobility/motor control drills to help those suffering back pain. If I can add in a relevant story about a frustrated patient that had a transformation, returning to full activity level, I create a much deeper connection with that audience.

One story I like to tell, particularly if I have a group with a lot of parents, is about one of our patients named Helena.

Helena is a mother of four and had been dealing with back pain for almost twenty years. She tried everything to resolve the issue—PT, chiropractic care, massage, and injections—but nothing touched it. She was sent to us by a massage therapy friend. Her main goal when coming to see us was not just to get her back to stop hurting but to be able to ski again.

Helena grew up in Sweden but had been living in the Atlanta area ever since college. She grew up skiing, and her kids were old enough now that she wanted them to start learning how to ski. Obviously, there's not a lot of snow in Atlanta, so they had planned a trip out to Colorado.

When I saw her, she wanted nothing more than to go skiing with her kids. She wanted them to love the sport she grew up loving so much. The problem was, she couldn't even pick up light objects without her back hurting. When we saw her, she was obviously frustrated and worried that she wouldn't be able to ski on the trip.

We saw her for about two months before her trip. The first day on the mountain, she held up great; in fact, she had zero restrictions the entire trip. She sent me a picture of her skiing while on the trip and thanked me for helping her share this experience with her kids. It's people like Helena that make me thankful to be a PT. I'm grateful to make a living in a way that gives people true long-term changes and creates a positive impact on their lives. It's incredibly rewarding.

Now, when I tell this story at a back pain clinic, I instantly create a bond with anyone who's had kids. It could be the mom, or maybe it's a dad who has seen his wife struggle with postpartum issues. They instantly make a link between what we were able to achieve for Helena and what we might be able to do for them or their spouse.

You might not remember everything from this book, but I bet you'll remember Helena trying to ski with her kids. Stories are so powerful, and picking a relevant story for the audience you are teaching is one of the most important ways to build trust and get actual patients from workshops.

The way you structure a workshop is also very important. We've found a simple framework that's repeatable, and it consistently converts patients.

Here's the framework:

- Intro/Inform on topic of the workshop (5–10 min)
- Teach a movement you'll test and retest (5 min)
- Teach a technique (5 min)
- Do the technique (5 min)
- Retest (1–2 min)
- Teach a technique (5 min)
- Do the technique (5 min)
- Retest (1–2 min)
- Teach a technique (5 min)
- Do the technique (5 min)
- Retest (1–2 min)
- Wrap up/pitch (5 min)
- Answer questions afterward

At this point, I've run well over 100 workshops. We've tweaked this workshop flow multiple times, and this is the one we've found to be the most consistent and repeatable.

There are a few key reasons you would want to set up your workshops like this.

The first reason is people get bored easily. Think about the last time you went to a workshop or a clinic. If the person leading it talked for more than ten minutes, you started to lose interest. The workshops you'll remember the most are the ones that involve a lot of hands-on work.

You want to make sure you start by educating participants on what they're learning and why. After that, you have to get people moving and interacting.

I've found the most success with MobilityWOD-style techniques. These can involve simple things like lacrosse balls or jump stretch bands. In particular, the lacrosse ball is something the attendees can leave with or easily get hold of to do the exercises at home.

The second reason is this allows people to see changes during the workshop. These are called *intrasession changes* and can make the difference between someone raving about you or not.

Here's an example. One of my favorite things to do is have people test and retest a forward bend. This one movement can be limited by a lot of things. I then have the attendees step on a lacrosse ball and move it around under their foot for about a minute on each side. Then we retest the forward bend. I've seen people improve their forward bend by 6–12 inches just with this one drill. That is a powerful intrasession change.

Intrasession changes develop trust and position you as the subject matter expert. No one likes delayed gratification but that's what we are selling with physical therapy. It's hard work, it can be uncomfortable, and it can take months to see true long-term changes. These intrasession changes give them a little win; and, even better, they got that change by doing something to themselves. How empowering is that?

Lastly, you want to take the time to close the workshop and position yourself as someone who can help them.

When I first started, I was terrible at finishing workshops. I would get nervous and basically just tell people, "Thanks for coming tonight. If you have any questions, I'll hang around." I never took the opportunity to effectively pitch myself or my practice.

Now when I run workshops, the last five minutes are really effective and important.

First, you want to summarize what participants learned and why it's important. After that, I tell them we'll be emailing video links for the exercises we went over. This sets the stage for them looking forward to an email and opening it.

Next, I position our clinic as a solution to their problem. I talk about how we help people get back to the activities they love and learn how to take care of themselves long term. I refer back to the relevant patient story I used in the workshop. Think about Helena's story. This is a perfect time to bring Helena back up and talk about how we help people like her.

Lastly, I transition people not to booking a visit but to talking with me afterward. I've tested this, and we get a significantly higher conversion percentage when people talk to us about their individual problems afterward. Make sure you let people know you're going to stay to answer everyone's questions. It's also important to let them know the questions don't have to be about them. It can be about their kid, spouse, or parent.

The number of questions you get after a workshop is a direct reflection of how well you were able to connect with people during that event. I've had some workshops where I've stayed for an hour afterward just answering questions. We get a lot of new patients from workshops like that. If you only have one or two people come up to you afterward, you're probably not going to get a ton of new patients from that workshop. Something was off. It could have been the content, delivery, or message. You have to keep practicing and tracking how successful these events are.

If you can get these workshops nailed down, you can build a practice off of it just like I did.

Part 3: Following up afterward

You've put in all the hard work setting up a workshop and you've finally run the event. Ten to fifteen people showed up, and you had a handful of people come up to you afterward with questions. One of those people called you to book a visit the next day. Success! New patient generation from a workshop. Many people will stop here. But if you don't follow up with people after the workshop, you're leaving money on the table.

For well over a year, I didn't follow up with people via email after a workshop. Looking back, I see I could have gotten a lot more new patients from workshops than I was converting at the time.

Typically, we will get about 10–20% of the workshop to convert to a new patient within about a week after a workshop. You'll get another 10% that come in or refer their friend or spouse over the next two to three months. I've even had people come in a year after attending a workshop. This is rare, but it definitely happens.

To double the number of new patients you get from workshops, you have to follow up with them via email afterward.

To start with, this can be as simple as an email with video links to the exercises you taught that night. They don't even have to be your own videos. If they are public on YouTube, they are fair game to share. Obviously, your own videos are even better, but if you haven't yet created content, don't let that stop you from following up with attendees.

The next step would be to set up an email drip sequence that automatically sends out emails afterward. These sequences can be great if you teach the same or similar workshop topics at different locations.

Let's say you have a workshop on improving the squat. You'll probably teach similar exercises at each of these workshops. To make it easier on yourself, create one email that has all the links to the exercises you usually teach at squat workshops. This will be the first email you send out.

After that, you can create a sequence of emails that goes out over the next one to twelve months, depending on how many emails you want to put together. We typically have email drip sequences that go on for two to three months for people who attend workshops. Here's a visual representation of what this drip sequence looks like:

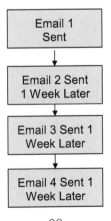

These emails are not sent from your personal email. You have to use an email provider that you can upload emails into and set up these automated sequences. There are a lot of options out there like Mailchimp and ConvertKit.

It doesn't really matter which one you pick as long as you start following up with people after workshops.

The framework you want to use is about one email every week for two to three months. After that, you can space it out to an email every two weeks. These need to be relevant to the topic of the workshop and have a call to action to either talk to you or book an appointment.

The other type of email that's very helpful is patient stories. You can set up these automated emails to mix in a few patient stories about people who have gotten really good results. The more someone can see themselves getting the result they want with you, the more likely they are to come in and see you.

The follow-up is crucial and will help you make all the time and energy you're putting into workshops worth it.

CHAPTER 16

CONTENT

The second part of our marketing pyramid is creating content. This content can come in a number of different forms. It could be blog posts, videos, newsletters, podcasts, infographics, or books. The entire purpose of the content we put together is to be helpful. We want to help people with free resources. We know that if we can help them or teach them something valuable with a free resource, they are much more likely to want to work with us.

Helping others and asking for nothing in return is a very effective way of building a bond and earning trust. As much as we want someone to land on our website and one minute later decide to become a new patient, that doesn't really ever happen.

You also have to understand that you're selling something no one really wants. "Oh, I really hope I have to go to physical therapy this year," said no one ever. People typically only see us when pain or dysfunction has gotten so bad they don't have any other options. What we do also requires delayed gratification. People have to come see us, work on limitations, and get some uncomfortable manual therapy done to them. To get the long-term outcome they're looking for can require months of work. This is a hard thing to sell.

We have found really high-quality content to be part of the decision-making process with many of our new patients. This could mean they view a video we created and posted on Facebook. It could mean they read a blog post that one of their friends shared. They might even have found their way onto our newsletter and were exposed to some content in the email that moved them to want to book a visit.

Really good content is the most effective way we've found to build trust with complete strangers.

Now, you might be asking yourself what content you should produce. This is an answer that I expect to change, but at the time of writing this, I would have you focus on blog posts and videos. The two work very well together and allow you to cater to different types of learning styles.

Before you start knocking out a bunch of content, I want you to look back at your niche and ideal customer. Your content should be focused on helping this niche and ideal customer deal with common problems. You want to write posts and record video with this one person in mind. The more you can talk directly to them, the more effective your content will be.

Before I even started seeing patients at Athletes' Potential, I started putting together videos and blog posts. I put out one video and one blog post each week for about two months before opening my practice. I actually enjoyed the process, and it was nice getting some of my thoughts out.

I vividly remember submitting my first blog post to be published on my website. I seriously was so nervous that my hands were shaking. It's an odd thing to put your opinions out in content at first. You worry that people will think you're an idiot and want nothing to do with you. Obviously, this doesn't happen even if your content sucks. It's still nerve racking to put your content out. It's normal, and it's something you just have to get over.

I also remember when I realized I was putting content together for the wrong audience. I noticed this after a few months of regularly writing blogs and putting out videos. On the blogs in particular, I started getting some comments. Most of them were positive, some of them were not. On one blog post, titled "The 4 Keys to Picking the Right Physical Therapist," I got a ton of comments. I also got people tweeting me, emailing me, and texting me about it. I thought this was great—I finally had a viral piece of content. The problem was, the only people reaching out to me were other PTs!

The content I was putting out was great content for PTs to read, but it was bad content for my potential clients to read. *I was educating and connecting with the wrong people.* It took me months to realize this, and it was a big lesson learned my first year in business. If you focus on putting together content for your ideal client, you'll avoid this big mistake I made.

Videos are the other type of content we have found to be extremely effective with cash physical therapy clients. Very few things allow you to connect with others as well as video does. Just think about how you like to consume content. If you're anything like me, you head to YouTube to look something up and you get sidetracked. An hour later you're still there watching videos of cats wearing birthday hats.

A perfect example of the power of video is Kelly Starrett and MobilityWOD. If you haven't watched the original MWOD videos, you should absolutely do it. Kelly decided to do a video a day for a year on movement/mobility. He recorded these videos on an iPhone, he didn't edit them, and he never did more than one take. They weren't the best quality videos, but the content was amazing. After a few months, the video project started picking up steam. More people shared the videos, and they got hundreds of thousands of views per video.

This one content platform catapulted Kelly into international speaking, multiple books, online courses, physical products, digital courses, and a very successful cash physical therapy practice/gym. That's the power of great content.

The biggest mistake people make with content is targeting the wrong ideal client, like I did early on with my content. The second biggest mistake people make is lack of consistency.

It is so common for people to start out making content and be really excited about it for a month. After that month, it starts to wear on them. They've exhausted all the topics they wanted to talk about, and now they have to think outside the box. They also get stressed out by the deadline of having to put together a blog post and/or video every week. Lack of consistency with your content will ruin your effectiveness.

The best way we have found to stay consistent with content is through batching. Batching content is where we schedule a time to do a number of videos or blogs at the same time. The best example of this would be scheduling a time to record videos. When we batch times to do videos, it's usually to create four to six videos in one session. That means we'll come up with what we want to talk about, who's going to do the video, and how it's going to be shot before we all get together to record. This prep work on the front end allows us to be really efficient when we do record our content.

If you properly batch your videos, you can get a month of videos done in about an hour. Now you still have to upload them, maybe edit a little bit, and share on your social media channels. These are minor tasks that an admin or a freelancer can help you with. What you can't outsource is the creation of the content. That has to be you or your other PTs.

The whole point of batching tasks like this is that it allows you to get in a deep work state. This deep work state is where you get to concentrate on one single task for an extended period of time. This allows you to be more productive as well as creative when you only have to focus on one task.

The other important aspect of a solid content strategy is a schedule. You don't want to be reactive with the content you produce. This is probably where many of you live. Does this sound like you?

"Oh shit, it's Friday. I haven't written a blog post or made a video yet. What the hell am I going to write about?"

If that sounds like you, you're living in a reactive state. This is a bad place to be, and it can significantly decrease the effectiveness of your content.

Try to work on staying one month ahead of your content schedule. If you put out one blog post a month, try and have four ready to go so you're not scrambling to write a post last minute. Using a simple content calendar like you see below is a great way to stay organized.

Blog Topic	Video Topic	Publication Week	Team Member
Back Pain Causes	How To Hinge	17 September 2018	Jake
Back Pain Options	How To Brace	24 September 2018	Danny

When you organize your content, try and pick a blog post and video that complement each other. You can even embed a video in your blog post. You also want to assign a date for this project to be completed and assign it to a specific person, identifying who will be in charge of putting together the content.

This is the basic structure of how we produce content at Athletes' Potential. It's something we go over every week at our staff meeting and make sure everyone knows what content they owe as well as when it's due.

The final reason to develop a solid content strategy in your business is to be able to use it in your newsletter. By newsletter, I mean a weekly email newsletter from your practice. This is an incredibly important step in our content strategy. Every month we get five to ten previous patients that come back in to see us as a *direct result* of these emails.

It's not enough to produce content. You have to share it effectively to get the maximum benefit of all your hard work on that content. A newsletter gives you a platform to share your content in a 100% non-salesy way. This is just an opportunity to say, "Hey, I wrote this cool blog and put together this cool video. Check it out if you're interested." Repetition and consistency are key with this. Our newsletter goes out every Thursday at noon. People know when it goes out, and they have become conditioned to seeing my name in their inbox once a week.

The content is not always relevant to every person on our email list. It's not about that; it's about keeping my name in their inbox on a regular basis. Also, sometimes the content you write is exactly what they're looking for. This is why we get so many patients coming back in because of content they read in the newsletter. We also get a lot of word-of-mouth referrals from content in our newsletters.

For example, let's say an old patient on our newsletter sees our email, and it's all about resolving shoulder pain with pull-ups. He may not be having an issue with it, but his friend recently told him he couldn't do pull-ups anymore because it hurt his shoulder. Our old patient forwarded our newsletter to his friend and told him to read it. His friend read it, liked what we had to say, checked us out online, and potentially ended up coming in to work with us.

Scenarios like this are how we consistently get 40+ new patients a month. It's not one big thing that we do that makes all the difference. It's a combination of a few marketing techniques and being very consistent with those techniques. We want a slow but consistent stream of new patients heading into our clinic by optimizing the three areas of local reputation, content, and digital ads. We'll talk more about digital ads in the next chapter.

CHAPTER 17

DIGITAL ADS

Imagine that cultivating a strong local presence and creating high-quality content is like building a little fire. The strong local presence is the kindling, and the content is the small fire logs you place on top. If you were a pyromaniac as a kid, like I was, you've probably squirted some lighter fluid on a few fires. Digital marketing is your lighter fluid, and if properly utilized, it can light your practice on fire in a really good way!

Before we dig deep into this topic, I want to set the stage for a second. The goal of this chapter is not to show you step by step how to create a Facebook ad or Google ad. In a couple years, these platforms can and probably will change dramatically. The components that won't change are how to get your message across with digital ads and when to use them. Let's get into how and why you want to add this element to your marketing strategy.

Let's use our perfect client avatar, Greg, for this example. We know Greg is a forty-eight-year-old male who is married, has two kids, is an attorney, and likes sports. We also know what zip code he lives in and approximately how much money he makes. Because we know all of this information, we can pay to have an ad placed in front of him on a number of different platforms. These platforms include Google, Facebook, YouTube, Yelp, Twitter, Instagram, Pinterest, LinkedIn, and a whole host of other platforms I won't even mention at this time.

Of these platforms, the two you currently want to focus on are Google and Facebook. These are the two most powerful for a few reasons. First, they are the largest and most active platforms on the planet.

Shit, Google is so big it's turned itself into a verb! How often do you tell people to "Google it"? You know you're powerful when you get to that level.

Facebook, on the other hand, is HUGE. The estimated user base in the US alone is approximately 200–250 million people. That means 60–70% of the entire US population are active users of Facebook. How would you like to get your brand and message in front of 60–70% or more of the entire population in your area? You can do that with Facebook ads.

As powerful as these platforms are, they will not make or break your local practice the way the first two parts of our marketing pyramid will. Digital ads are designed to be stacked on top of a really solid reputation and consistent, high-quality content. If you have the base and the middle of the pyramid in place, digital ads can literally change the trajectory of your business.

There are a few powerful ways to utilize digital ads. My current favorite ways to use them are as follows:

1. Building content bridges
2. Retargeting
3. Direct search lead generation

Building Content Bridges

In the content section, we talked about how different types of content are great at developing trust. The picture below will give you a visual representation of this. Our goal with content is not to get them all the way across the bridge. The goal is just to get them to take the first few steps across the bridge. It's a way to develop trust and build a bond.

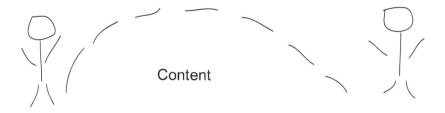

Content

There are three types of traffic you can work with using digital ads. The first type of traffic is what's called cold traffic.

Cold traffic is basically people who don't know who you are or what you offer. This is the biggest group of potential clients out there.

The second group is called *warm traffic*. These are people who have been exposed to your business in some way. This could be via word of mouth, having consumed some of your content or just stumbled across something to do with your business online. This is the second largest group of potential clients.

The third group is called *hot traffic*. These are people who know who you are and know you have a service that can help them. This may be someone who calls your office after their friend tells them they have to work with you. This may also be someone who leaves you a contact request form and they are actively asking you to reach out to them. This is the smallest group of potential clients but the most likely to work with you in the short term.

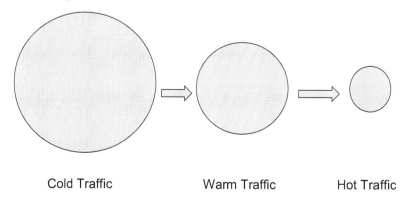

Cold Traffic   Warm Traffic   Hot Traffic

The problem with most business owners is they want to make the sale right away, so they only focus on the hot traffic. Look at the picture above for a visual representation of this. Imagine only focusing on this tiny circle that represents the hot traffic. You're going to miss out on the huge potential client base in both the cold traffic and the warm traffic.

The reason most business owners just focus on the hot traffic is because it can be difficult to work with cold and warm traffic audiences. You cannot use the same marketing strategy with cold/warm audiences as you do with the hot traffic audience. The best approach we have found is to try to move people from one type of traffic to the next. By this I mean moving them from cold to warm and warm to hot. If you try to turn a cold prospect into a hot prospect overnight, you're going to have a difficult time successfully using digital ads in your practice.

This is where you can really leverage all of the content you've been working so hard on. This is the perfect first step of the bridge to get someone from cold traffic to warm traffic.

Imagine you're a forty-five-year-old female dealing with a tennis elbow issue. You play in a tennis league with your friends. You're not super competitive, but you have three kids, and this tennis league is how you get some adult conversations in your life and stay sane.

You're on Facebook one day and you see a sponsored video in your news feed titled, "The Top 3 Exercises to Alleviate Tennis Elbow." It's enough to get you to stop scrolling and looking at videos of cats wearing birthday hats (yes, this is the second birthday hat cat reference). You test out a couple of these exercises and notice you get some temporary relief in your elbow. Finally, some hope that this will resolve! You get busy and head off to do the twenty other things on your to-do list for the day.

In this scenario, we have successfully moved this person from cold traffic to warm traffic. We've shown her that we can help her without seeing her or laying a hand on her. That's a pretty powerful thing, and it's a great way to build goodwill and trust. The more goodwill you build, the more people will move from cold traffic to warm traffic. The more warm traffic you cultivate, the higher likelihood you have of turning warm traffic into hot traffic, which eventually become clients.

Here's what you *don't* want to do with cold traffic.

Let's take the same cold traffic scenario of the forty-five-year-old female with tennis elbow. You decide to put a video ad in front of this person. In that video, you describe all of your credentials and how long you've been a physical therapist, and you explain why people watching this video should come and work with you. This would be equivalent to you going up to some stranger in a bar and asking them to marry you. You're moving too fast. You've got to at least buy them a drink first. Putting a relevant piece of content in front of someone is the PT lead generation equivalent of buying them a drink.

Once you've taken cold traffic and turned it into warm traffic with relevant content, you can change your messaging. These warm leads are now people familiar with you and your brand. Retargeting these people with another step to build more trust is the best approach.

First, let's explain retargeting. I'm going to get a little techy, so don't fall asleep on me.

Have you ever wondered why when you go to Rogue Fitness to look at barbells, you see ads for barbells everywhere you go? Well, Rogue is smart, and they sell a shitload of barbells. This basic marketing strategy is called *retargeting* or *remarketing*.

This can occur because Rogue has a piece of code on their website called a *pixel*. This pixel basically follows you around the Internet after you land on a website. Facebook and Google currently do this better than anyone. Facebook also allows you to track people who watch videos of yours or go to your page on Facebook. This allows you to build actual audiences of warm leads that you can then work to move along your marketing continuum to eventually become hot leads.

I'm not going to get into how to install a Facebook or Google Analytics code on your site. A simple YouTube search will come with thousands of videos showing you how to do this. The real importance of this is that you want to understand when and why you want to use it.

Retargeting these warm audiences allows you to get more specific about what you're offering them. One classic example of this is an ebook.

An ebook, by the way, is just a larger piece of content that has been packaged into a PDF. It's basically a mini book on a certain topic. It's really designed for you to trade something in exchange for a prospective client's contact information.

Let's say you have a blog post on drills that runners can do to improve their warm-ups. If you place a pixel on your site, you can track the people who have visited. Now you can create an ad to be placed in front of these people online, offering to send them a free ebook. To get the book, they just have to opt in by putting in their name, email, and maybe a phone number. This is a common lead generation tool, and it allows you to reach these prospects via email or phone.

This allows you to be very specific about what information these people are interested in. The more relevant content you can put in front of the right people, the more likely it is they will turn into patients.

The strategy we prefer to use at Athletes' Potential is to try and drive warm traffic to a contact form. We offer free fifteen-minute phone consultations with our docs for anyone who wants it. In order to sign up for one of these, you have to fill out a contact form that gives us more information.

We get information like how long you've had this injury, how you heard about us, the details of your current injury, if you've seen any other providers, and your basic contact information.

Over the past few years, we've had about an 80% conversion rate with people who submit a contact form. That means eight out of ten contact forms we get turn into patients. This is huge for us in terms of predicting new patient volume. Much of our digital marketing efforts are focused on driving warm traffic to turn into contact request leads. Once they have submitted a contact request, they turn into hot traffic.

Another form of hot traffic is inbound phone calls. This is where someone typically looks you up online and decides to call about your services. This search engine is usually Google. It's one of the reasons Google Adwords can be very effective.

Now, go back and look at the marketing pyramid before you go spending $1,000 a month on Google Ads. If you don't have a solid reputation, it's less likely that these people will call you. You also need someone to answer the phone. Every time you miss a phone call, you're losing out on a potential new customer. If you don't have administrative infrastructure, this type of paid marketing can be ineffective.

Being able to talk to and convert these new leads into patients is one of the keys to success in this model. Don't worry, we'll go into depth on phone skills and phone selling later in this book.

Here's the biggest takeaway from this chapter: Understand what type of traffic you are working with. Is it cold, warm, or hot? From there, move those people along the continuum of going from cold to warm and warm to hot. Put the right message in front of the right people at the right time.

Most importantly, stop asking someone you just met to marry you.

SECTION 3:

SALES

CHAPTER 18

MINDSET

The most important persuasion tool you have in your entire arsenal is integrity.
—Zig Ziglar

When people hear sales, they instantly think about that bad experience they had at a high-pressure car dealership. We've all been there. You just want to look at a car, and next thing you know, you're there for two hours, sitting in different rooms and talking to different people's bosses. It left you with a bad taste in your mouth, and you've hated the idea of sales ever since.

On the flip side, we've all been to an Apple store. You walk in and someone asks you if you need help with anything. You say no and then immediately take your kid over to the kids iPad area so he can be distracted while your wife is in Lululemon trying on yoga pants. While you're in there, you start looking around and see the new watch they just came out with. You walk over, check it out, and another store associate comes by. They let you know a little bit about the watch and answer your tech questions about it being able to track your running distance. Your wife comes strolling in, yoga pants in hand right as you're getting your new Apple Watch. Your kid is still getting his mind melted by Fruit Ninja. You've just been sold to in a completely different way.

Sales doesn't have to be a bad thing. In fact, if you do it right, it doesn't make your consumer feel bad at all. You think you left that Apple store regretting that you bought the watch? Hell no. You're probably putting it on as you walk out of the store!

Everyone hates being sold to with old-school high-pressure tactics.

Everyone loves to buy things—from a new car to a watch to physical therapy—*when sold the right way.*

In this section, I'll go over what I've learned about sales. Some of this comes from courses and training I've done. Most of this comes from interacting with thousands of customers in my practice over the past few years. I cannot overstate the importance of rock solid sales in your practice. In a cash practice in particular, we cannot afford to be wrong as often as a big in-network corporate-owned practice. We have significantly less room for error, but when done the right way, effective sales will be a huge part of the growth of your practice. And it starts with cultivating the right mindset.

Mindset is an interesting topic. It can mean different things to different people. You can talk about mindset in regard to sports, business, or life in general. In this context, we will talk about how it applies to your business. To me, mindset is how you truly feel about the service or product you're selling. It's a deep internal confidence, or lack of confidence, associated with what you're doing in business.

You can't fake having the right mindset. You can absolutely work on this like any other skill, though; you can develop an improved mindset when it comes to business. Some of this can be planned, and sometimes events just happen that change the way you view things.

I definitely had difficulty with selling myself as a physical therapist that didn't take insurance when I first started Athletes' Potential. When people asked me about insurance, I would almost get defensive. I responded this way because I was frustrated; I lacked the confidence to directly state what I charge and really feel its absolute value to everyone I worked with.

This all changed after a conversation I had with my accountant in early 2015.

My accountant was a patient of mine, coming in to see me about some elbow pain he was having. This elbow pain was referring from his neck, and over the course of about six weeks he made a full recovery. He was sitting in my office at his last visit, and he said to me, "Danny, you're not charging enough money."

Now, that's an odd thing to hear from an accountant. They are notoriously frugal, and it shocked me when he said this. At the time, I was charging $175 a visit, and I thought that was way higher than I should be charging.

He said, "Danny, when I first came in here, I thought I needed elbow surgery. This is the fifth time I've seen you, and I have no elbow pain. Even better, I feel stronger than I have in years, and I've got way more energy at the office. You're not charging enough for what you help people do."

That conversation helped me make a really important mindset change about how I viewed my services and accepted money for them. My confidence level when talking to people about what I did skyrocketed. Our revenue also dramatically improved after that conversation and the mindset shift I made.

What had happened was a true internal change in how I viewed what I was worth. I went from thinking what I did was too expensive for all but ultra-rich people, to believing what I did was an absolute bargain compared to the alternatives.

Think about this. According to Medicare data, the average MRI in the US costs $2,611. What actual benefit comes from that MRI? In most cases, absolutely nothing. In fact, you can have more false positive findings from an MRI than actual beneficial information. Even at our current rate of $200 a visit, we would have to see someone thirteen times to equal the average cost of an MRI! Thirteen visits with my company is a downright bargain compared to getting an MRI.

Look, as PTs we help people in so many amazing ways. You have to see it from the lens of my accountant. He has no problem charging people $350 an hour to do tax prep. Why do we have such a hard time charging even $150 for a PT visit?

It all comes down to your mindset. It's based on the value you're providing, not the money you're charging. You also need to look at the alternatives. People spend years avoiding activities they love because of pain or fear of injury. People get needless surgeries, and they feel no better after the surgery than they did before. We are in the middle of a pain medicine epidemic, and it's largely due to people in pain searching for a solution.

Why can't that solution be you? We see little miracles every day when people get back to running after years of avoiding it. We see people go from being dependent on others to becoming self-sufficient and feeling empowered. We see people avoid surgeries they were told they absolutely had to have.

Take a step back and realize what you're capable of. Realize how important you are in the healthcare landscape and to the people you directly help. It's your obligation to see what you do as amazing. This will change your mindset in its own right. You'll start viewing yourself as a solution and an advocate for the patients you work with. You also have to accept the fact that what you do is valuable.

It's okay to accept money for doing something that helps others. It's not a bad thing to make money. Think of how many amazing things you can do with that money.

You can build a company that provides amazing jobs to amazing people like we have done. You can support the non-profit organizations of your choice. You can build true wealth and financial security for yourself and your family. You can experience the world in ways many people can't because they lack financial security.

Your practice will start out with just one person: you. That person will dictate the growth of the entire company going forward. You will dictate how well your company handles success and failure. You will develop the culture and the why behind what you're doing. The more clarity you gain on how important your work is, the better mindset you'll have to handle the inevitable difficulties that come with owning a business.

Just remember the advice I once got from entrepreneur and author Jesse Itzler. He told me, "Money is good for three things. It's fun to make, it's fun to spend, and it's even more fun to give away."

You decide how much impact you get to have, and as scary as that might sound, it's also amazing.

CHAPTER 19

YOUR RELATIONSHIP WITH MONEY

Most people think that money will make them happy,
but in reality it's a happy life that makes you more money.
—Jim Fortin

Money is an interesting thing. Most people have a very poor relationship with money. They think if they could just win the lottery, all their problems would go away. They view it simply as something that buys you other things. Most people also think that all they need is to make some more money to be happy. If you are going into business for yourself, you need to take a step back and reevaluate your relationship with money.

As a kid, I was always fascinated with money. My family wasn't poor by any stretch. We were about as middle class as they come. My dad was in the Army, and my mom stayed at home with my brother, my sister, and me. We always had everything we needed but not necessarily everything we wanted. We were taught that hard work gets you things but also that you want to work smart, not necessarily hard. I always wanted more and was constantly trying to sell things to my siblings and friends.

When I was ten years old, I found a *Hustler* tucked into a hole in a tree in the woods. I was walking our family dog, Daisy, and that particular day she decided to pee on a tree that just so happened to have this magazine tucked into it. Seriously, as a ten-year-old kid, this was better than hitting the lottery!

What happened next might surprise you and prove my theory that sometimes we turn into entrepreneurs, but more often we are just wired to be entrepreneurial.

After taking the magazine home, I sat down and tried to decide what to do with it. I knew I had to show my friends. This was a big deal, so I had to get the word out. Before I did that, I had an epiphany. I realized this was valuable, really valuable. Right then and there, I decided to sell it.

As I sat there deciding my best course of action, I realized that even my richest ten-year-old friends would only probably be able to pull together $5 for this treasure I had found. I also thought that each of them already had a dollar or could easily find one.

That night while everyone was sleeping, I took a pair of scissors and cut out pictures from the magazine. When I was done, I had about fifty individual pictures and decided that the next day, the *Hustler* sale would start at Pinckney Elementary School.

My first day in business went really well. I sold about ten pictures, mostly in the bathroom, but also a couple on the playground after school. The next day was even better. I sold the remaining forty pictures. In two days, I had made $50 off a magazine I just happened to find in the woods.

Now, before I lose you, I tell you this story because this was my very first taste of true sales, supply/demand, and placing a value on something. I would have to work for hours in the yard pulling weeds, cutting the grass, edging, and picking up leaves to get a couple dollars in allowance. Here in the span of a few hours of selling, I made more money than I had ever seen in my life. My world had been turned upside down, and I realized it wasn't about working harder—it was about working smarter.

This is something my dad always said. His dad, who died when I was very young, lived by this idea of working smarter. He always had a side hustle going on. Even when he was in the Air Force during

World War II, he was running dice games on the side to make a little extra money to send to my grandma.

The other thing my parents did that I'm very grateful for is get me physically difficult jobs. I honestly think my dad went out of his way sometimes to find the worst jobs for a teenager to do. My brother and I did things like working at Christmas tree lots in the winter and shoveling gravel with prison release workers for a heating and cooling company over the summer. Worst of all was detailing cars at the Goo Goo Car Wash in the blistering summer heat of Columbus, Georgia.

This is the second time I've referenced the Goo Goo Car Wash, so it must be obvious that this place left an impression on me. There's nothing worse than breathing in tire shine while some guy sitting in a chair with a mist fan points out how many spots I need to redo. These jobs taught me an appreciation for hard work and dealing with people of varying backgrounds. It also gave me a strong desire to not have to do this type of work for a living.

Here's the thing about hard work that's important to understand: Hard work doesn't necessarily equal more money. In fact, many people who work the hardest get paid the least for their efforts.

Most people think you just have to work hard and everything will pan out for you. Well, I can tell you the men I shoveled gravel and washed cars with worked really hard. They also made very little money. They were always struggling and asking for pay advances from our bosses. If hard work equals more money, why didn't these men make more?

Now I look at some of my entrepreneur friends, and I see some of the wealthiest people I know working fewer hours. One friend in particular has a music company. He works about four to eight hours a week on this company, and he makes more money than almost anyone I know.

Now, he didn't work four to eight hours his entire career. He busted his ass starting his company and worked 60+ hours for years. He did this with intention. He did this with the goal of building a company around him. He didn't just work hard every day without looking at what he was working on. He worked in a smart manner for those first years to set in place the infrastructure to be able to step back from the grueling work schedule required to start the company.

So, hard work doesn't necessarily equal more money. For some of you, that might be a hard paradigm shift to make. You may also have a handful of other false beliefs when it comes to money. Here are a few:

- Rich people are evil.
- More money more problems.
- Why should I charge for helping people? I feel guilty charging people for PT services.
- Wanting money and charging people cash for PT is greedy.
- I don't deserve to charge money for PT.

Why do we have these false beliefs? What did your parents teach you about money? For many of you, they probably didn't teach you anything. You more than likely just learned about money through the actions your parents took with money.

If you are in business or going into business for yourself, you must have a healthy relationship with money. How can you expect to charge someone $200 for a visit with you if in your head all you're thinking is, *This is way too much money. This person can't afford it.*

I had this very problem when I started my practice. I literally thought no one could afford to pay me for my services. I would feel guilty telling people what I charged, and I would discharge people as quickly as possible so they wouldn't have to pay too much money.

I didn't value what I did as much as my patients valued the service they were receiving.

At the time, I had a belief that there was just a finite amount of money and no one had enough to afford my services. I couldn't have been more wrong, but this was a very difficult mental hurdle for me to get over. Like many of you, I love working with people as a physical therapist. I love helping people get back to physical activities, and I enjoy watching them improve at each visit. I get a ton of personal satisfaction from this process. I would do it for free the rest of my life if I didn't have to pay a mortgage or feed my family.

The idea that people can't afford you or they are going to spend their grocery money on a PT visit is ridiculous. What people do with their money is their decision. I can't think of many things that have a better value than spending an hour with a high-quality practitioner.

The last issue with money that new PT entrepreneurs run into is what they should do with it after they make it. The traditional mindset is that you make money to buy something else. Now this may be true in a way, but money needs to be used for much more than that.

Think back to my friend in the music business that I referenced earlier. He paid himself a modest income for years in his business. Even after starting to make really good money in the business, he still paid himself just what he needed for his family to live a comfortable life. What was he doing with the rest of that money? He was using it to build.

You see, money is a tool to acquire assets—not just to buy things you need. What I mean by that is, money is a tool to get things that either get your time back or make you more money. This could be in a traditional sense like a stock or a mutual fund. You buy this asset, which pays you a return or dividend, and that money grows. If you buy a slightly bigger TV, it earns you no more money; and, in fact, that TV will depreciate in value very quickly.

When we look at this through the lens of a clinic owner, money allows you to grow your company. Assets in the company are things like technology that increases what you can charge or adds an additional revenue stream to your business. It also includes people and building your main power infrastructure.

I recently wrapped up a consulting project with a two-clinician cash-based clinic here in the US. These two PTs are swamped with patients, which is a good thing. When I initially talked to them, they wanted my help getting more new patients. As we continued to talk, I realized that they were doing everything themselves and didn't even have an administrative team member. That meant they were putting together all the superbills, scheduling and rescheduling everyone, responding to every email, returning every call, and mailing all their bills off themselves. They were making good money, but they were time poor.

These tasks are $15-an-hour tasks. It doesn't take a DPT to be able to do these things. In this scenario, the clinic charged about $200 a visit. That means for every hour of admin tasks they performed, they were losing $185 compared to what they could make seeing a patient.

They viewed this admin staff as a cost, not as an asset. True, this person isn't a direct revenue-producing employee. This person is what I like to call a force multiplier. This is a person who allows your key clinical staff to do their job and focus solely on generating revenue as a clinician. This admin person is a huge asset and directly frees up your time to do many other things that drive your business forward.

You have to look at money as a tool to acquire more assets to grow your business. If you take home everything you make and spend it on a wakeboard boat, you're an idiot. You'll never even be able to use the boat. You'll always be working in your business, doing tasks that a number of other people can do just as well, if not better than you.

Leveraging money into infrastructure in your business does two things: It creates an actual, true business—the kind of business that allows you to step away while it still generates revenue. It also creates time freedom. This may be the most difficult and elusive quality of becoming a business owner. The freedom to dictate what you do, when you do it, and how much of it you do in your business is a place very few people get. Using the revenue you do make to build a team is the only way forward for a local service business like a cash practice.

Build a team, invest in those people through extensive training, and you'll eventually have both financial and time freedom.

CHAPTER 20

THE PSYCHOLOGY OF SELLING

I vividly remember the first patient I saw at Athletes' Potential. His name was Sam, and he was a defense contractor who lived in Birmingham, Alabama. He had been emailing me for weeks about getting in to see me. When he first emailed me, the main problem was I didn't even have a business yet. I was still in the Army. I had no office for Athletes' Potential, but I had been writing blog content for a few months. He had seen a blog post I wrote on shoulder issues and had decided I was the person that could finally help him with a slew of musculoskeletal health problems he was having.

Finally, on day one of Athletes' Potential opening up, Sam was added to the schedule. That day was June 9, 2014. He asked me how many visits he could be seen in one day since he was coming in from out of town. I didn't know what to tell him because I didn't have anyone else scheduled that day. I told him I could see him from 10 a.m. until 12 p.m. but I had some other appointment after that (which I didn't). He wanted to be seen at least three hours, so we agreed on him being seen from 9 a.m. until 12 p.m. The day he showed up, I had no idea what the heck I was going to do with this guy for three hours. I had never worked with someone for three hours straight before. Turns out, he had a ton of movement issues from decades as a police officer and now as a defense contractor. We went over everything I could think of for three hours in the gym. I was mentally exhausted, and he was physically exhausted by the time we were done. My visit rate was $175 at the time, and we had discussed this on the phone. When we were done with the three-hour block, we went back to the office, and he asked me if I took cash. I honestly didn't know if we could accept cash, but I said yes because I figured that was better than saying, "I don't know." What happened next changed my view on our business forever.

Sam pulled out exactly $525 in cash and put it on the table. I didn't even count it because I thought that might be rude and would look unprofessional. I stood up, and he gave me a big sweaty hug. He thanked me for my time and for teaching him how to take care of his body. He left, got in his truck, and drove back to Alabama.

I went back in my office and sat there for a few minutes. Eventually, I picked up the cash and counted it. Sure enough, it was $525 exactly. I had never been paid for physical therapy before. I especially had never been paid in cash for physical therapy. It's hard to describe, but I think that first patient paying cash was one of the most important things that happened to me. It wouldn't have been significant if he had paid with a card. Cash is something you can see and feel, and even though it's just paper, you know it has value.

After I finished counting the money, I stood up, threw the bills on the desk, and said, "Fuck insurance … I'm never dealing with that shit!" (Hence the title of this book.)

This is the moment I knew Athletes' Potential would work. The other thing I realized was that I felt really good about myself after that time with Sam. I felt like I'd given him a ton of really important things to prolong his career and improve his current physical state. He saw value in that and was more than happy to pay me for that time. The selling of this also felt very easy and natural. It didn't feel like selling at all. It just felt like a conversation between two people who agreed that this service was worth this amount of money, and that was it.

I had always been told that sales is dirty. Sales is what used car salesmen use to get you to buy a piece-of-shit car. It's what telemarketers do when they talk elderly people into buying some crap they're selling over the phone. I had just had a $525 sale that felt totally natural and effortless. I didn't feel bad about it at all and, in fact, the guy who paid me had even given me a hug on the way out the door. *Sales doesn't have to be sleazy.* In fact, it shouldn't be, it should be effortless like it was with Sam, and there are some factors that can lead to this effortless approach to selling.

Also keep in mind that the ability to sell is a skill. Skills can be developed, and they require practice.

One of my first business mentors told me a tale of two lumberjacks.

Lumberjack A cuts wood all day. Lumberjack B cuts wood as well but keeps stopping and sitting down throughout the day. At the end of the day, Lumberjack B has four times as much wood cut as Lumberjack A. Lumberjack A asks: "How could you have cut so much more wood than me? I saw you stop and rest multiple times today." Lumberjack B says: "I wasn't resting. I was sharpening my axe."

Practice sharpens your axe. This is true with your clinical set, but it's also very true with sales. We have staff meetings every Thursday for two hours at our office. At least half of that time is going over sales scenarios for our PTs and our admin team. That's how important sales is to our business. You have to keep sharpening the axe.

I alluded to factors that can make sales easier. Factors that can make selling seem effortless. We'll dive into each of these factors below in more detail throughout this chapter:

- Establishing Trust
- Pre-framing
- Future-framing
- Reciprocity

- Social Proof
- Authority
- Likeability
- Commitment and Consistency
- Scarcity

Much of the basics of these concepts are drawn from research and books written by Robert Cialdini. He has written many amazing books. Two of my favorites are: *Influence* and *Pre-Suasion*. I also want to give credit to the books written by Daniel Pink, Jeffrey Gitomer, and Neil Rackham. I did not come up with these concepts, but I do want to specify how they can be used in our profession. If this topic interests you, make sure to read the work of these authors.

Establishing Trust

Establishing trust seems like it would be obvious in regard to better selling. The more someone trusts you, the more likely they are to do business with you. This is very true in regard to any type of clinical work.

People are trusting you with their most important asset, their bodies. In most cases they aren't 100% sure what you do or what you're going to do to them. The more you can establish trust before they come in, while they're in your office, and after they leave your office, the more likely they will be to comply with your recommendations.

The following sections will feed into the ability to establish trust. This will make or break your ability to sell.

Pre-Framing

Pre-framing is one of the best ways to establish trust. Pre-framing is basically explaining the next steps in a process to someone and telling them what they can expect. Here's an example.

When we have a new patient, they get an email from our team that explains a few things. First, we welcome them to the Athletes' Potential community. We let them know where the office is located and how to get in touch with us if they need to reschedule or if they get lost.

We also let them know what to expect during the visit to take the anxiety of the unknown out of the equation.

Here's an example of a welcome email.

Fred, thanks for booking a visit with Dr. Jackie. We're all excited to help you get rid of your back pain and get back to [insert whatever activity he said he wanted to get back to].

Here are a couple things to know before you show up for your visit.

First, you should have gotten our online waiver/forms via email. If you haven't, please let us know.

We also pride ourselves on being punctual and not making you wait to be seen. If your appointment is at 9 a.m., you'll be seen by the doctor at 9 a.m. We only have two chairs in the waiting area, and they're not comfortable. You won't be sitting in them very long.

Please wear something comfortable that you can move in. You won't be working out or doing anything that will make you sore. All of our doctors are experts in evaluating movements, so we'll need you to wear something you would wear to go running or to the gym. This allows our doctors to see what your movements look like without having to battle restrictive clothing.

At the first visit, the doctors may or may not do hands-on treatment. It depends on what they find and what you feel comfortable with. Just because all of our doctors are certified in dry needling doesn't mean you're going to have needles put in your body during this appointment.

At this visit you'll get a few things. First, you'll gain a clear understanding of exactly why you're having these issues. Next, you'll get customized homework that's specific to solving your problem. We do not practice cookie-cutter medicine here.

You will also have clear channels of communication with your doctor during the entire process. If you have a question after you leave, you'll get a timely response from your doctor to address it.

If you have any other questions, please let us know by emailing us back at this address or calling us at [insert number].

We look forward to seeing you and helping you get back to [insert whatever activity he said he wanted to get back to].

Respectfully,
The Athletes' Potential Team

Pre-framing is built into this email all over the place. Any time you're subconsciously answering a question, you're increasing trust. For instance, we have gotten a lot of potential new patients that ask if they will get needles put in them at the first visit. We do a lot of dry needling, but we don't use it with everyone. We have become known for this, and it's a good thing. Some patients with a fear of needles want to make sure that's not going to happen. On the phone, and again in this welcome email, we pre-frame that they are in charge of what happens.

We also pre-frame that we are on time. How many times have you gone to the doctor's office and been forced to wait thirty minutes or even an hour to be called back for your appointment? You show up on time, but they waste an hour of your day while you read about this season's pies in *Southern Living*.

We pre-frame that they will not be waiting. We literally only have two chairs, and they are very uncomfortable on purpose. People do not wait at our office. They are seen on time, every time they have an appointment.

Pre-framing is an incredibly powerful tool allowing you to quickly build trust with your clients.

Future-Framing

Future-framing is another incredibly powerful tool in sales. Some people actually do this all the time without realizing it. These are the visionary people who are very future biased. They are the ones willing to put money away now because they can visualize what their future will look like if they invest early. These are the people with big dreams that tell other people all about them. The big dreamers are the ones people want to follow because not everyone naturally dreams about what could be.

Dreaming is just future-framing. When we do it with our patients, we help them see what life can look like once their problem is resolved. Here's a good example from a patient I saw the other day. He used to exercise five days a week, but over the past few years, he's fallen into terrible shape. He has pain in his knees, shoulders, and back. He's lost a good bit of muscle and is frustrated, to say the least. The problem is, he's an entrepreneur and works a crazy number of hours. He's sacrificed his body to build a software company he recently sold. Now all he wants is to be pain free and be able to exercise again.

I put a general movement program together for him, and one of the movements was push-ups with his hands on a bench. This is an easier version of push-ups, and I had him do them until he couldn't hold perfect form anymore. He did nine push-ups. After he was done, he sat on the ground and said, "This is so sad ... I used to be able to do forty actual push-ups without stopping."

Here's what I told him: "I know this sucks right now, but there's only one way to get past this. You have to follow this plan and commit to getting stronger. In two months, this elevated push-up will be so easy, it won't even be worth your time. You'll be doing much harder movements by then. For now, this is where we're at. If you commit to doing the work, you'll get back to exercising just like you used to, and you'll be pain free."

Now we may say things like this to our patients all the time, but I said this intentionally. I wanted to future-frame for him what would be possible in just a short period of time. Bringing up a movement he was struggling with and future-framing how much easier it would be allowed him to see what's possible. When we have patients who are in a bad place like this guy, future-framing can make the difference between sticking with it and giving up. It's also the difference between them dropping off our schedule and finishing the visits in the plan of care we develop.

Reciprocity

Ever wonder why those nice ladies at Costco hand out so many free samples of tacos, crackers, and cheese sticks? Behind that inviting smile is a sales ninja in disguise.

Research has shown that offering free samples can increase the likelihood of someone buying a product by up to 30%. Costco is smart, and those samples may be free, but they serve a purpose.

When someone does something for you or gives you something, you feel a strong desire to give back. This is a deeply rooted desire to reciprocate, and it works well as a sales tactic. We can use this same sales principle in our clinics in a number of different ways.

First, you could use something like a free ebook, video series, or phone consult as a giveaway. This is the PT equivalent of dangling a taco in front of people like Costco does. Even something as insignificant as a video series can have a major impact in terms of reciprocity.

Taking this to another level would be sending people individualized self-work. We do this as part of our front desk sales sequence. If our admin team has a prospective customer on the phone and they aren't ready to book a visit, we send them one or two videos that we feel will be beneficial. This has helped us save a ton of patients that otherwise would have moved on to the next PT practice that probably was in-network with their insurance company. We are giving them something of value that can help them. As a result, they are much more likely to want to reciprocate by coming in to see us.

Lastly, this can also be used with networking. When I first meet someone, they almost have to fight me to pay for the lunch or coffee. Yes, I'm a nice guy, but I also understand reciprocity. Even that $4 latte gives me an advantage when it comes to this principle. Reciprocity is huge, and it works.

Social Proof

This is a concept that belongs in both the marketing and sales sections. *Social proof* is the idea that the opinions of others mean more than what you say about yourself.

Think about what you typically do when you buy something on Amazon. Let's say you're buying protein powder. You type "protein powder" in the search bar and get a list of thousands of protein powders that you could purchase. You probably look at the name of the company, the price, and the packaging, but most likely the reviews are what grab your attention.

Let's say you were buying this protein powder and you started looking at the number of reviews each option had. Let's say one option has 100 reviews, another option has 50 reviews, and the last option has 1,000 reviews. Which one are you most likely to pick? I don't know about you, but I'm going with the protein powder with 1,000 reviews.

This is social proof in a digital context, but the same principle applies for services like PT. We have review options out there, and people look at them. The main two right now are Facebook and Google. Most prospective clients will read these reviews when making a decision. If you don't have any reviews, you're less likely to get picked. If you have a whole bunch of reviews, you're more likely to get picked.

People want to do business with providers who have already been vetted. This could be via a word-of-mouth recommendation or a digital search where reviews play a big part. If you don't have reviews, start collecting them now.

Authority

We all have degrees on the wall, and that inherently gives us authority. Once someone is in the office, they can see your diploma and know you at least have the degree your website said you have.

Authority can be much more powerful than that now, especially with content. Creating content is something that gives us a platform. It also gives us perceived authority. Here's an example.

A couple years ago, three USC DPT students started an Instagram account called The Prehab Guys. They started making videos of things they were learning in school and on their clinical rotation. They also started putting videos out on exercises they were doing at the gym. Because of these consistent and helpful videos, their platform grew and grew. As I write this book, they have around 350,000 followers on Instagram. I had the opportunity to talk to them on the Doc and Jock Podcast a couple years ago. They were smart for sure, but I can't say they were smarter than a lot of bright students I've had a chance to talk to.

This is the entire point of authority: You don't have to be a bestselling author anymore. You can build your own platform by consistently putting out high-quality content in a niche where you can provide value. The Prehab Guys did it and executed it flawlessly. I'm sure they've received more business opportunities from their success with this single platform than most students coming out of school. Authority is something that can be earned in a much shorter period of time now than even ten years ago.

You don't have to become an authority on prehab exercises like The Prehab Guys did. You could decide that you want to be the authority in your local market for runners. The same principles apply. Pick a platform, stick to it, and consistently put out really good content.

The platform could be Instagram, Facebook, YouTube, a blog, or a podcast. I'm honestly not even going to name any more platforms because in ten years there will be different ones. It's not about the platform, it's about finding your voice and being consistent with the platform you choose.

You can become the go-to expert in any area if you follow this framework. You just have to position yourself as an authority, and eventually you'll become the authority.

Likeability

It may sound like it's not fair, but people do business with people they like. It's been that way forever, and it's not going to change. Let's talk about how to get people to like you more. I don't know about you, but this sure would have been helpful when I was in middle school.

There are a few factors you can use to your advantage when it comes to getting people to like you more.

First, is appearance. I'm not telling you to go buy a whole bunch of new clothes. What I mean by this is people like you more if you look more like them.

Here's a good example. If you were going to meet a CrossFit coach at their gym, would you wear a suit to that meeting or shorts and a T-shirt? If you picked shorts and a T-shirt, you'll have a much better likelihood of that person wanting to do business with you. The reason is you look like him. It also shows that you understand the culture of the gym.

We can also do things like modeling. This is where you mimic the body language of the person you're talking to. The first time I tried this, I almost laughed out loud. I felt like it was so obvious, but it's not. People have no idea you're modeling them unless they have learned about modeling. Now we're getting into weird *Inception* dream-with-in-a-dream territory. Let's leave it at this. If your body language looks a lot like the body language of the person you're working with, they'll like you more.

Sharing similar interests can also be a huge factor in someone liking you. This is a common technique used by car salesmen. They're taught to look at the car someone shows up in and try to create a similar interest. I have an Army sticker on my car, and so does my wife. Every time we've ever been to a car dealership, they bring up the military very quickly. It's either that they were in the military or their brother is in the military. Either way, they are trying to establish similar interests by bringing up the military.

The same thing works with our patients. If they come in wearing a shirt from a golf course, it's easy to bring up golf. If you golf and that person golfs, all of a sudden you're talking about who won the Masters, and you've created a deeper connection. This can be a really effective way of gaining likeability.

Commitment and Consistency

This is another one of those deeply rooted tribal behaviors. Back in the day when you and I were walking around looking for berries and hunting deer, we did so in a tribe. One of the worst things you could do in a tribe is lose the trust of the others. Because of this, people would almost always stick to their commitment and be consistent, fulfilling what they say they're going to do. If you lost the trust of the others, you could be kicked out of the tribe. That meant getting eaten by a bear, and that's not a good way to go out.

We also have a very strong desire to be consistent and follow through on commitments. We all know people who say one thing and then do something else. You probably don't trust these people too much. We don't want to be those people, so we do what we say we're going to do.

Your patients are no different. In fact, if you do a good job of getting small commitments from them, they are more likely to make a big commitment to you.

Ask questions like:

Are you going to do your exercises twice a day like we talked about? Yes.

Are you committed to resolving this back pain for good even if it takes a few months? Yes.

When they say yes, they're more likely to actually do it. If they told you they were willing to commit to solving this back pain issue but then bailed after two visits, that's inconsistent. They have committed to you, and they are much more likely to fulfill that commitment.

Make sure you're asking people questions that challenge their commitment and consistency. This will get you better outcomes and more people to finish your plan of care.

Scarcity

Scarcity might be the greatest sales principle of them all. The reason is that most people are procrastinators. They will not take action unless they have to. When they feel like they are going to miss out on something, all of a sudden they have a reason to act.

So how do you structure scarcity into your practice? First, you can start by not being as available. I was told to do this before opening up my practice. It was actually great advice, and it helped me convert patients early on. Instead of opening my schedule five days a week, I only opened it two days. Only having those two days gave people a sense of scarcity in my schedule. They were more willing to come in and work with me and more likely to work around my schedule.

You can also have limited-time offers for initial services. Let's say you teach a workshop and offer the attendees 50% off their first visit. It would be even better if you made this offer expire after seven days. If you send emails to people letting them know they're going to miss out on the 50% off evaluation, you'll get a lot more people taking you up on that offer.

Scarcity is real, and it's incredibly powerful. It can't be fake scarcity either. You can't say one thing and do another. You have to follow through on the scarcity you're layering into your practice. If you can do this, your sales will increase and so will your revenue.

All of these principles are useful, but let's bring it all together. Let's do it using the example of answering the dreaded "do you take my insurance" question. In the next chapter, we'll cover exactly that.

CHAPTER 21

SO ... DO YOU TAKE MY INSURANCE?

In one way or another, I've always had an association with the military. Three of my four grandparents, both of my parents, my brother, and my sister-in-law have all served in the military. Both my parents were enlisted in the Air Force, and eventually my dad moved over to the Army while my mom stayed home with me and my two siblings.

I tell you this because there are some really interesting aspects to your life when you grow up on a military base. Seeing tanks and Humvees driving around is about as normal to Army kids as seeing a street sweeper is to civilian kids. Watching groups of soldiers in formation running around early in the morning chanting cadences about jumping out of airplanes was our entertainment while we waited on the bus.

The last aspect of growing up on a military base that's unique is that the healthcare system is completely free. This socialized medical system definitely has its pros and cons. Free healthcare for my parents with three kids constantly ending up in the emergency room was probably a huge blessing. What paid for healthcare wasn't money, though; it was your time. It was also a typical lack of continuity with your provider.

I can't remember ever going back for a checkup or a sick visit and actually seeing the same physician. Customer service typically wasn't the best either, but the care was free, so it didn't have to be.

Need a checkup? You owe $0.

Have a baby? You owe $0.

Need a lifesaving surgery and have to stay in the hospital for a month? You owe $0.

I was covered by the military's healthcare from the time I was born until I finished college. I never had an insurance card, paid a copay, or needed to figure out coinsurance/deductible. If I was sick or got hurt, I just whipped out my military dependent ID card and I was good to go.

After college I went straight into the Army, and the cycle of being covered by military healthcare continued. This time I wasn't a dependent; I was actively serving myself. And I got to see the inner workings of the system from the provider side as well because I was going into the Army to become a physical therapist.

Again, in this system I never charged anyone for care, checked benefits, or issued superbills. If a patient's back was hurt, they just came to see me. Now, it might take them three weeks to get a new patient evaluation appointment. I may not be able to get them back for a follow-up visit for a month either.

There are some incredibly smart and capable medical professionals in the military healthcare system. The challenge for them is to function within a system that is understaffed and has tons of red tape involved. My exposure to this system of healthcare is one of the main reasons I decided to go the cash physical therapy route when I opened Athletes' Potential.

In a strange way, my lack of traditional insurance experience was beneficial. On one hand, I was used to doing my job for a salary but never really associated that with billed units I sent off for approval to a healthcare system. On the other hand, I had never accepted money for providing physical therapy to people.

My mindset about insurance was basically: "Hey, I don't know a whole lot about your insurance, but if you want to work with me, this is what it costs."

Now, this isn't the most intelligent or sophisticated way to handle questions about taking people's insurance. Surprisingly, though, this approach worked pretty well. I definitely had an advantage with timing too. Over the past decade or so, deductibles have risen, and people are required to pay more for their healthcare. This actually makes my type of clinic a much more viable option for the general population.

My mindset and ability to communicate with patients about insurance has evolved quite a bit. We've tried to keep it as simple as possible because we have other staff members who are also expected to answer the question, "Do you take my insurance?"

Over the years, we've tested different ways of answering this inevitable question. If you're a cash practitioner, you probably die inside a little bit every time someone asks you if you take their insurance.

We now answer this question with three additional questions, in particular with inbound phone calls.

It typically goes like this:

Caller: Caller: Hey, I was calling because I've hurt my knee, and I saw you guys have a lot of good reviews online. I just wanted to call and see if you take my insurance.

Staff: Hey, thanks so much for calling. I can help you with this. The answer to your question is a little more complex than a yes/no question. Do you mind if I get some more information from you first to help better answer that?

Caller: Caller: Sure.

Staff: Great. First, my name is Claire. Do you mind if I ask your name and **why you're seeking help for this injury now?**

The first part of this is to move from a direct yes/no question to getting their info and figuring out why they're calling you. The simple answer would be, "No, we are not in-network with your insurance company." But we know it's more complex than that.

They may have a $3,000 deductible that hasn't been met. They are 100% out-of-pocket no matter where they go. They may also have met all of their deductibles and get 50–80% back from their insurance company with a superbill. These are all things you do not want to tell them in the first minute of starting your relationship. Get their information and start figuring out why they are calling you.

This question—Why are you seeking help for this injury?—helps you figure out what is driving this person. People are procrastinators. It's human nature to put things off until you're either running out of time or getting so uncomfortable you have to do something about it. Just think about when you were in college. You knew you had a paper due in two weeks. Why not finish that paper on day one and be stress free for the next two weeks? No one does that. We all waited until the night before and scrambled to put together a half-ass paper on the rise and fall of the Byzantine Empire. Our patients are procrastinators as well. Figure out why they are calling. This answer is not just knee pain, by the way, it's more than that.

Caller: I'm calling now because my knee has been bugging me, and it's stopping me from running.

Staff: Oh, do you run a lot? And are you training for anything in particular?

Caller: Caller: No, I run when I go to Orange Theory, and now it's gotten so bad I've had to stop going.

Staff: Staff: That sucks. Orange Theory is a great workout. Have you been training at Orange Theory for anything in particular?

Caller: Caller: Well, I'm getting married in about six months, so I've been going so I can lose a little bit of weight before the wedding.

Staff: Staff: Oh, congratulations! Where are you getting married? (This conversation could go on for a couple minutes about wedding details, but it's a big part of connecting with the caller.)

This is where the gold is. Someone will go see a physical therapist because their knee hurts. Someone will drive across a state to see a physical therapist if that person can help get them back in the gym so they can lose weight, feel more confident, and be proud of their wedding pictures for life. This goal of losing weight before the wedding is what we will reference with the person the rest of the conversation.

Next, figure out the answer to the following questions: Where are they now? And where do they want to be?

Staff: So, from a physical standpoint, how much weight are you trying to lose before your wedding date?

Caller: I'd love to be about 10–15 pounds down from where I am right now. I'm just frustrated because if I can't work out, I don't think I'm going to be able to lose that weight.

Staff: I totally get it. I do CrossFit, and I've hurt my knee before. It completely stopped me from being able to work out. I was actually worried I might need surgery, but the docs here got my knee back to 100%, and I haven't had to avoid working out at all.

The third part is to let them sell themselves. You want to ask why they think you are the right fit for them.

Staff: So, one last question. Why do you feel our clinic is the right fit to help you with this problem?

Caller: Well, I looked at a bunch of different clinics on Google, and you guys had a ton of good reviews. I started looking at your Instagram page, and it looks like you guys deal with a lot of athletes. I think this clinic is a good spot for what I'm dealing with.

Staff: We definitely see a lot of athletes and a lot of people looking to get back to working out. It can be really frustrating to try and do the right things like work out and eat well but get sidelined by an injury. We help people just like you every day get back to working out pain free. We can definitely help you get back to Orange Theory so you can stay on track to lose the weight you want before your wedding.

This is the end of the third part of our structure. Now we will explain the specifics of our clinic, offer to check out the caller's benefits, book them for an eval, and send a helpful video to continue to build rapport.

Staff: Now to get back to your insurance question. We are what's considered an out-of-network clinic. That means we don't have any direct contracts with insurance, and that's a really good thing for you. All of our docs make decisions based on what's best for *you*. They spend a full hour with you every time you come in, and we have complete transparency about what you pay. You won't get one of those frustrating bills from us three months later for $500 like you will from most doctors.

Our fee is anywhere from $179 to $199 a visit, depending on if you decide to do single visits or purchase a package with us.

Now, a good percentage of our patients do get reimbursed by their insurance companies for visits with us. It really depends on if you've met your deductible and what your benefits are. I'd be happy to check that for you and give you a clear picture of what you can expect to potentially get reimbursed. Would you like me to do that?

Caller: Yes, that would be great. Insurance is so confusing. It would be amazing if you could check that for me.

Staff: No problem. In the meantime, let's do this—let's get you scheduled for an evaluation with one of our docs. Their schedules book up quickly, so let's at least get a visit on the books while we check your insurance. I'm also going to send you a video our team put together on some basic knee pain self-treatment exercises you can start doing at home. This will give you something to work on until you get in for your evaluation.

This last part of closing the visit is really important. We want to do a few things. First, we want to let the caller know we are transparent about being out-of-network and want to help them better understand what they can expect with their insurance. This will be helpful no matter if they end up working with us or a different PT clinic. Second, we want to get them on the schedule. This dramatically increases the likelihood they will come in for a visit. Last, we want to continue to foster goodwill by sending them a helpful video that also lets them see members of our clinical staff. If you don't have an admin team, it's up to you to do all of this. I know that sounds daunting, but it's much better than having no new patients.

This same approach is used with outbound calls from people who have expressed interest in working with you. This could be via a contact form on your website, a Facebook or Instagram message, or an email referral from a past patient.

The whole goal is to engage with someone on the phone in these three basic areas:

1. Figure out why they are actually looking for help.
2. Let them verbalize where they are and where they want to be.
3. Let them tell you why they think you're the right fit.

If you can get this down, it can change your clinic forever. Ethically and effectively answering the insurance question is one of the most important things you need to work on as a cash practitioner. Keep it simple so you can train admin members on how to do this and you'll be on your way to gaining time freedom from many of the tasks you really shouldn't be doing. Never lose sight of the fact that you have to be able to teach others how to answer this question in order to scale. If it's just you doing everything, you will make good money but be time poor. You need others in order to build a true business and impact more people. Start thinking of all the tasks you do through the lens of a business owner, not just someone who is self-employed.

CHAPTER 22

THE THREE-PART CLINICIAN SALES PROCESS

It's the moment of truth. All of your hard work marketing and getting out in the community has paid off. Sitting in front of you in your office is a new patient you know you can help. You know your clinical skill set is good enough to help this person get a full recovery. The challenge is, will they finish their plan of care? Will they come back after their pain is gone? Will they commit to you to get the change they are looking for? This is where an effective in-clinic sales process will save the day.

I use a three-part sales process with new patients. This is the same process I teach to all of our staff PTs as well. Here's what I want you to remember:

- Question
- Shift
- Solve

Question

The first part of this process is to question people about why they are actually in your office. This should have happened on the phone already, and I encourage you to review the previous chapter if you haven't read that yet.

We want to follow a very similar structure of questioning people on why they are coming to see us. I like to use kids as an example.

I have a five-year-old daughter named Maggie. She's in that stage where she asks me all kinds of "why" questions. The other day she asked me, "Daddy, why is it raining?" I don't know anything about weather, so I responded, "Well, the clouds are just heavy, Maggie." She replied, "Why are the clouds heavy?" I responded, "Because they are full of water." She replied, "Why are they full of water?" I responded, "I don't know. Let's just ask Mommy when we get home."

Obviously I know nothing about rain or weather. When it comes to sales, though, this exchange illustrates how questions can be powerful.

Typically, we are taught to ask people about their goals. We ask people what goal they have for physical therapy. This usually leads them to tell us some physical goal they want to be able to achieve. It could be getting back to running, sleeping through the night without pain, or throwing a ball again.

We typically stop there, write down the goal, and move on to the mechanism of injury and ease/agg factors. As important as those things might be, you are losing a golden opportunity if you don't ask a follow-in why question.

For instance, let's say the patient has a goal of being able to throw a ball.

One additional why question could lead you to a true internal reason for why that person is in your office.

You might ask, "Why is throwing a ball so important to you?"

He might respond, "Because I'm coaching my son's baseball team this year, and I don't want to have to rely on other parents to throw batting practice."

This helps us drill down to the internal reason he's in our office. The external reason would be his shoulder hurts when he throws a ball. The internal reason would be that he wants to be able to throw batting practice to his son and his teammates. He also doesn't want to have to rely on other parents and be a burden on them if he can't throw.

If you just talk to this person about their shoulder pain, they will come in for two visits and leave after they have decreased symptoms. If you get this person talking about throwing a ball to his son and not having to rely on other parents, he'll see you as many visits as needed to resolve the issue.

Imagine you're a five-year-old asking why questions, and you'll get to the real reason patients are coming into your office.

Shift

The next step in the sales process is where we shift a patient's perspective and help break false beliefs. This is about building trust, and sales really does rely on the act of developing trust with another person. If they trust that you are the right person to solve their problem, they'll happily pay you to solve it.

The way we shift their perspective is with a relevant patient example. In the next chapter, I'll go deep into how we structure our patient stories, but for now I'm going to show you the basics of where this fits in the evaluation.

These relevant patient examples can be interjected into your evaluation at multiple points. You can even use multiple patient examples. Let's take the example of the dad trying to throw without pain.

You have a couple options, and the one you pick depends on that person's personality. For instance, if this patient was once an athlete and is a big sports fan, I would bring up the NFL and MLB players we have worked with to solve shoulder pain.

If he wasn't a big sports fan, I would bring up a relevant patient that was as similar to his presentation as possible. Ideally, it would be someone struggling with shoulder pain when throwing, someone who also has kids.

We want to paint a picture for them of the processes that similar patient went through. From being frustrated, to finding us, to following a plan and, finally, to achieving the goal they were after. If you can interject a relevant patient story, you can get that patient future-framing his own recovery. This allows him to essentially daydream about the process and the result he is trying to achieve.

Our whole goal here is to help the client believe that their goal is possible. It's also to assure them that they don't need more invasive medical care like injections, surgery, or imaging. If you can set their mind at ease and stack that with a relevant patient story, you'll shift their belief.

Solve

This is the last part of the in-clinic sales process, and it's where it all comes together. This is also the part where people typically have the hardest time. This is primarily due to the fact that you are going to have to confidently state your recommendation and ask for a commitment from the patient.

This phase of the sales process happens at the very end. The goal of this phase is to summarize what they have told you, explain the diagnosis/prognosis, and offer a solution.

The first part of this is reciting the internal reason for why they came to your office today. If it's because they want to throw a ball to their son and don't want to be a burden on other parents, you need to say that. You basically need to repeat back to them what they told you. After you recite this, you need to ask them if that's right.

This is important because you want to start creating what we call micro-commitments. This is basically where someone commits to you on a very small level. They are stating that you're right about something or that they are willing to do something. This makes them much more likely to commit to your plan.

After that, you want to give a definitive prognosis of how many visits you expect to see them. If it's ten visits, tell them that. If it's six, tell them that. You're an expert, so act like one. Our staff like to talk about all the people we've helped, relating a relevant patient story, and explain that we typically see a problem like theirs for X number of visits.

It's also important that you pre-frame the fact that you fully expect pain to be resolved in a fairly short period of time. You also need to pre-frame the fact that pain going away doesn't equal the problem being solved. This will dramatically help with your drop-offs.

From here you have two options: You can offer them the package options for visits that you might have at the evaluation. If you think the client is a no-brainer, offer it to them. If you think the client needs a bit more time or isn't quite as sold on you, hold off until the second visit.

This second visit package offer can be very effective. The patient gets a chance to see how your process works, they typically come back feeling better, and they are much more motivated to commit to you on the second visit.

Either way, you need to give them a way to commit to you, and a package does that. It allows you to get the positive cash flow of up-front payments as well as a true commitment from the patient. For the patient, they get better results because they are fully bought in on what you are doing.

You have to be confident, and you have to tell them your honest expert opinion about what they can expect. The more you can confidently tell people what they need, the more people you will get to commit to you.

Also, don't forget to interject relevant patient examples in this first visit or two. Those stories help people see themselves going through the same process. It's incredibly powerful, and we will spend the entire next chapter talking about how to structure these stories effectively.

CHAPTER 23

THE POWER OF STORIES

Everyone loves a good story. My wife is reading the *Harry Potter* books to my daughter right now, and she loves it. Actually, my whole family loves it. Ashley and Maggie sit on the bed reading the book. Jack and I lay on the carpet with our dog, Buster, listening to every word. We get sucked in, and time flies when we're listening to a story or watching a story (a movie or a show) on TV.

Researchers estimate that the human mind spends about 30% of the day daydreaming. I would say it was more like 50% for me when I was in school. I was constantly daydreaming about other things I wanted to be doing. Those daydreams are stories in our mind.

Stories are one of the few things that can actually hold the attention of a human for longer than a few seconds. Especially now with social media and more content than you could ever consume available on your phone. It's harder and harder to get and keep people's attention. Stories are how we can do that. In particular, patient stories in your clinic.

This content belongs in both the sales and marketing chapters; stories are an incredibly effective marketing tool. Stories can also be used during the sales process to help customers see what's possible if they commit to working with you.

We tell a lot of stories in our practice, and we've found a framework that we follow as we deliver a story. This can be used in a video, an email, or even on your website. This is just a structured way to show what's possible when people commit to solving a problem and get some help from you along the way.

Here's the Patient Story Process:

- Introduce the patient.
- Introduce their problem/frustrations.
- Describe when you met them.
- Describe the plan you gave them.
- Describe the struggles and eventual success.
- Where are they now?
- What should people do next?

I'm going to use one of our patients we love to highlight for this example as I take you through the process. I'm going to tell you Helena's story.

Introduce the Patient

Like many of our patients, we first saw Helena when she was in a really bad place in her life. From the outside, she looked like she had a great life. She was happily married, had four healthy kids, and lived in a great area of Atlanta. She had grown up in Sweden and had been an athlete her entire life. She even skied on a national level as a youth athlete.

Introduce the Problem/Frustration

The problem was that Helena had been unable to stay injury free for the past decade. It started with some mild back pain, but over the years it got increasingly worse. It got so bad that she had to avoid picking her kids up from the ground. Every time she got one of her kids out of the bathtub, she hurt her back. Imagine being a parent who can't even get their own child out of the bathtub.

She had seen a number of different providers over the years. She had seen chiropractors, massage therapists, pain management doctors, and everything in between. The result was the same each

158

time—temporary relief and then a frustrating return of her pain and limitations.

Describe When You Met Them

Finally, her running partner convinced her to come see us. She was obviously frustrated and got very emotional talking about feeling like she was a burden on her husband. The fact that she couldn't do simple things like vacuuming or picking her kids up made her feel terrible.

When I got a chance to watch her move and evaluated her back, I realized that her back was fine. She was healthy, and nothing was damaged or broken. The problem was that she was using her back all wrong. You see, back pain is common but not normal. More often than not, it's caused by simple factors that compound as we continue to use our body inappropriately for years.

I explained to Helena that she didn't need surgery. She was in the right place, but I wasn't going to fix her. I was going to teach her how to fix herself.

Describe the Plan You Gave Them

When you've been to as many doctors as Helena has over the past decade, you're skeptical at best. She committed to giving this approach a chance and understood there would be work and challenges along the way. She also understood that I'd be there to help her at every step. We even set a goal. Helena had grown up skiing and still loved to ski but had avoided it for the past ten years. She was fearful of hurting her back while skiing. The goal she set was to take her entire family on a ski trip and be able to introduce her favorite sport to her kids.

Describe the Struggles and Eventual Success

The first huge step for Helena was when she realized that how she moved affected how her back felt. Primarily, this meant how she picked things up. When we first got started, she was fearful of even picking up a 20-pound kettlebell. I showed her how to load her hip instead of her back when she picked things up, and all of a sudden, she had no pain picking up a 20-pound kettlebell. Her face lit up like a Christmas tree when she did this. You seriously would have thought she'd just hit a home run. This simple movement change resonated with her and gave her confidence that she could get back to living a normal life.

Over the next six months, she had highs and lows. She vacuumed the house without pain for the first time in decades, but she also woke up with an aching back without knowing why. As she continued to follow the plan of moving better and getting stronger where she needed it, the good days started to outnumber the bad days.

In February of 2017, Helena took her family to Keystone, Colorado. She was nervous about the trip but was excited as well. She had made so much progress and was doing things she'd never done before. She was running pain free again, pushing a stroller, and even doing kettlebell swings in her garage with her husband.

I saw her when she got back from the trip, and she was so excited to show me all the pictures she'd taken. She skied for four days straight. She had a little bit of soreness after the first day but knew exactly how to take care of her body. She used the things she'd learned over the past six months and resolved her own soreness in a matter of a few minutes. The next three days were completely pain free, and she did everything her kids and her husband did. Best of all, she knew that her history of back pain wasn't going to hold her back from living her life anymore.

Where Are They Now?

I still see Helena occasionally. She drops in to say hello to me and our staff. More often, I see her around the neighborhood—running with her friends, a big smile on her face, and still pushing a stroller.

What Should People Do Next?

If you're frustrated and sick of avoiding things you love, we need to talk. It doesn't have to be that way. Helena spent a decade frustrated, scared to pick her kids up, and avoiding a sport she loved growing up. It doesn't have to be that way; we can help. Click the button below. Let us know a little bit more about you and what you're trying to accomplish. We'll match you up with one of our doctors to see if you're a good fit for what we do. If not, we'll help you find the right place to get the help you need. Stop avoiding life, and start living it again.

I lay this entire story out for you so you can see how we structure a patient story. You should also be able to see the power of how Helena's journey is explained. Imagine you're a person with kids, and you have lower back pain. Reading this story gives you hope. Reading this story gives you a hero—and that hero isn't me, it's Helena. You start to view the possibility that you can achieve the same thing.

This is what we want from a story. We want to give people hope and structure a daydream for them. We want to connect with them on a deep level.

There are two levels at which you can connect and communicate with people. The first level is *external*. In this case, that would be back pain. Back pain sucks, but plenty of people deal with back pain for decades and never seek help.

The second level is the *internal* level. In this case, that would be feeling like a burden on your family because you're limited by back pain. This is a level that will drive action. If you can connect and communicate on this level, people will seek your help. Not only that, they will be less price-sensitive and more committed to whatever solution you offer them.

Stories help us highlight the external problem but show that we also understand the internal problem. Stories are one of the most powerful marketing and sales techniques you can use.

This same story can be explained to a prospective patient over the phone. If they're skeptical about paying out of pocket to see us, a story like this can help get them to book a visit. This same story can be used in the clinic with a patient. This can help improve their compliance with both home exercises and completion of your plan of care.

Telling relevant stories during the first visit or two with a new patient significantly increases the likelihood that they won't drop off. These drop-offs will frustrate you, decrease your outcome effectiveness, and limit your business revenue.

Use this patient story framework to lay out a couple of your home run patients. Use them as often as you can. Teach them to your staff, and make sure to highlight that your patients are the heroes—you're just helping them along the way.

CHAPTER 24

CONTINUING THE RELATIONSHIP

I honestly think traditional physical therapy clinics have a terrible business model. We've been taught all through school and even when we get out of school that the goal is to discharge people. In the Army, we would try to get them in and discharge them as quickly as possible. Part of this was because of lack of man power. Part of this was because it was a metric tracked by the hospital. This discharge model is broken, and I learned why one day from a patient of mine trying to run a marathon in every state.

About two years ago, I started working with a female runner. She was a veteran runner and had a big goal. She wanted to run a marathon in all fifty states, while she was in her fifties. At the time, she was fifty-two. I thought this was an amazing goal, and I was excited to work with her.

She first came to see me because of a foot issue she was having. It was pretty straightforward, and I ended up seeing her about four times. On the fourth visit, I gave her some additional programming I wanted her to do and some recommendations for returning to running then I sent her on her way.

Two weeks later, she showed back up on my schedule. At the time, you could book yourself online, and that's exactly what she did. I was a bit confused and figured she might have had a re-aggravation. Her foot was actually fine. She was here to get some help with a hip that was notorious for flaring up when she started putting in longer miles.

I saw her another two visits for this issue, gave her some additional homework, and discharged her again. Two weeks later, there she was on my schedule again. At this point, I was starting to get a little frustrated. I was borderline obsessive about my average clinical rate, which was under three visits per person at the time. I didn't want her driving my average up.

At this visit, I asked her what was going on, and she said nothing was wrong, she just wanted to get me to watch her move and to work on whatever I thought needed work. Looking back, I almost can't believe how oblivious I was to the fact that this was my ideal patient. Someone who looked at things *proactively* instead of reactively.

I was a bit frustrated and explained to her that I help people fix their problems and teach them how to take care of themselves. I explained that I wasn't all that interested in maintenance work. What she said next changed my view of our business forever.

She said, "Danny, let me explain this clearly to you. I'm a fifty-two-year-old woman trying to run a marathon in every state over the next eight years. I don't have time for setbacks. I want to avoid them entirely. I like what you do. I would like to pay you to work with me on a more regular basis. If you don't want this work, give me a recommendation to someone who does."

I honestly felt like I was six years old again and my mom had just put me in time-out. This patient had just challenged me. She'd drawn a line in the sand: either you help me in this capacity or send me to someone else. I realized how silly this discharge mindset was, and the only reason I was doing it was I didn't know any better.

What my patient helped me realize was that a lot of our patients would love to be proactive instead of reactive. They are looking for someone like us to quarterback their health and wellness. I also realized how unique the skill set of a Performance PT actually is. Think about it. We can help people get out of pain, move better, feel better, *and* improve their performance in whatever sport they train for. Why are we discharging these people so quickly? We can add so much value to their life.

At this point, I started learning about continuity programs and the holy grail of business revenue: *recurring revenue.*

In our profession, a continuity program is just a structured service option for people to work with us on an ongoing basis. This could be in a lot of different variations. It could be an actual monthly visit going forward. It could be following a custom or general digital program. Honestly, it can be anything you think adds value to someone's life.

Recurring revenue is revenue you get every month without having to go out and find new business. It's predictable, stable, and has a high likelihood of being there every month. Increasing the amount of recurring revenue in your business will change your business forever. It's the most important type of revenue that we track, and here's why.

Instead of looking at the next month and thinking to yourself: *How/where am I going to find ten to twenty new patients? How many workshops do I need to do? How many networking events do I need to go to? How much money do I need to spend on advertising?* What if you had fifty visits on your schedule that were already booked. People who had committed to working with you in an ongoing manner. If your goal was to get 100 visits per month, half of those visits are already there.

This is the power of a continuity program that adds a recurring revenue stream to your business. If you're charging $200 a visit, those fifty visits would equal $10,000 in revenue. Half of your monthly revenue goal is met without you having to go out and find it. It stabilizes your schedule, gives your best clients a great option to be proactive, and adds a unique recurring revenue stream most other businesses would love to have.

The reality is, this type of continuity option is not appropriate for all of your patients. It is, however, appropriate for many of your patients. Let's do the math for a second.

Let's say you have ten new patient visits per month. Eight of those ten people would be a good fit for your continuity plan. If you get just 25% of those patients to commit to your continuity plan, that's two people added per month. The beauty of this type of plan is that it's compounding. It's not just two additional visits you're adding. It's two, plus an additional two on top of that every month going forward. Month one you have two people in the plan. If you sell it to two more the next month, you have four people in the plan. You'll have six the month after that, and so on and so forth. It grows, and as it grows, the number of new visits you need to find goes down.

If I could go back and tell myself anything when I started Athletes' Potential, it would be to give people a continuity plan option instead of just discharging everyone. At this point, we've seen well over 1,500 new patients in the city of Atlanta. Even moving 10% of those people over to a continuity program would give us 150 visits per month that we wouldn't have to go out and find. That's a lot of revenue and a lot of stability.

So how do you position this type of program? Well, it's something that needs to be sold along the way and not just at the very last visit. This is where we dive back into the sales principles of pre-framing and future-framing.

As we are working with a client, we'll bring up other similar patients who are like them and have moved to our continuity program. We'll pre-frame that this may be a really good option for them based on how they've responded to what we do and their goals going forward. This typically happens about halfway through the plan of care.

We also future-frame what they want their life to look like when they're older. We bring up the question of what they want to be able to do when they're eighty years old: *Do you want to be dependent on other people and physically limited, or do you want to be active and independent? Do you want to be moving around the world in a walker by that age, or do you want to be picking up grandkids and still working out at that age?*

This future-frame is really powerful and helps people realize the power of being preventive versus being reactive about their health.

Keep this in mind also: Your clients will stop buying from you for just two reasons.

Reason #1: You've offended or irritated them in some way. They no longer like or trust you at this point.

Reason #2: You've given them nothing else to buy.

In our profession, we rarely offend or irritate people. In many cases, we have the best relationship of any type of medical provider with the client. They like us, and we get to know them on a much more personal level than their primary care doc or their dentist.

That leaves only reason #2 for why people stop buying from you. You're just not giving them a reason to stick around. If they have nothing left to buy, they leave.

Keep this in mind as well: People are going to seek ongoing work somewhere. It's going to be from a personal trainer, massage therapist, chiropractor, or any slew of other health/wellness professionals. Why can't this be you? Is your skill set not good enough to function in this role? Of course it is. You just need to give these people the option.

Adding a continuity option on the back end of your service offerings will change your business. You'll also change a lot of lives in a very positive way. People need accountability, and they need help. The Performance PT is uniquely positioned to fill that gap.

CHAPTER 25

THE EASIEST SALE YOU CAN MAKE

Over the past few years, I've had an opportunity to work with hundreds of cash-based Performance PTs. Over and over again, I hear the same story. This might even sound a little like you.

You graduate from school thinking you are going to set the profession on fire. You get your first job at a corporate- or hospital-owned clinic. They promise to not have you see a massive schedule, but within six months you're seeing 20+ people a week.

You do your best to handle the volume and eventually fall into a groove at work. The problem is, you start to like your job less and less after about a year. You feel more like a waiter than a medical professional. You're constantly managing multiple patients at once, and you just don't have the time to do the detailed manual therapy or movement training you know could benefit these patients even more.

To make matters worse, the documentation is getting more complex, and you just got another questionnaire added by your supervisor that everyone has to fill out. Your lunch break is just a time for you to catch up on your notes. You have to stay after your last patient for thirty minutes to an hour just to finish up your notes. You're at the office for ten hours a day, and you really don't love what you're doing.

You wonder if all that time, effort, and money to get your degree was worth it. You start scouring the Internet for other options, and you stumble across something about cash physical therapy. You instantly go down the rabbit hole of learning everything possible about cash physical therapy.

Finally, you decide you have to make a change. You're not sure if the cash physical therapy route will work, but you just can't stand being in this PT mill job anymore. You find a little space in a local gym where you work out, and you start seeing people on the side.

Things start going well enough that you decide to jump ship and go full time at your dream of owning a cash-based Performance PT clinic. You realize quickly that people won't just show up at your office begging to book a new evaluation with you. Marketing and sales are challenging, so you look for a guide. This is where I typically get emailed, messaged, or called.

Here's the number one question I get: "Danny, how do I get more new patients?"

I always answer with a question: "How many prior patients have you seen?"

Here's why I care about this. Past patients are an untapped gold mine for most practices. Most practices do a terrible job of staying in touch with patients and continuing to have a relationship with them. They also stop giving them a reason to come back in the clinic.

In October of 2015, I decided to run my first patient reactivation campaign. I had recently read a book by Jay Abrams in which he made a very strong case for why you should prioritize your past customers. The truth is, this is the easiest group to sell to. All of these people already know, like, and trust you. They also have already paid to work with you and are much less price-sensitive.

I figured I would give it a try and, to my surprise, I was able to reactivate over $5,000 in prepaid packages in less than a week.

We've now run, upgraded, and improved this original campaign each year. It's gone from generating $5,000 in a week to generating

$80,000 in a week. Much of this is because we have more patients to reactivate at this point. If you've seen fifty to a hundred people, you should easily be able to reactivate 10% of your prior patients to buy a prepaid package.

We do this by crafting a compelling offer. There are a couple parts to creating an offer that people want to buy.

First, you want to keep it simple. Give people one, maybe two options. The more options you give them, the more you'll confuse them.

Next, stack other things of value on with your core offer. For instance, we offer a ten-visit package at a slight discount. We also stack on a training program that we put together for people to follow at home. The core offer is the package at a discount. The value stack to help them get a better result is access to a workout program written by our doctors.

Generating new patient leads is an important part of any clinic. Almost every clinic I've ever done consulting with has completely forgotten about their past patients. Before you go and spend a ton of time and energy on new patient lead generation, make sure you're optimizing your past patients. They will be the easiest sale and the most loyal customers. You just have to give them a reason to come back in.

CHAPTER 26

CONCLUSION: WHAT NEXT?

Well, that's it! We did it.

If you're anything like me, you probably skipped around this book. You might have jumped straight to this chapter. Don't worry, I do that all the time. Seriously, though, I wrote every single word of this book for you. If you're like me and you read the first ten pages and then skip to the conclusion, go back and read the entire book.

The information in this book is drawn from five years of being in the cash-based PT trenches. It's also drawn from the hundreds of other practice owners I've worked with along the way. This book wasn't written to be some kind of fable to teach you a lesson about life. This book was written as a field manual to help you become a success. Use it as a field manual. Reference it if you need to figure out how workshops should be run. Use it if you are having trouble selling your services to your clients. This is the intent of this book.

I also realize all this information can be overwhelming. If you're wondering what to start with first, here's what I recommend:

- First, if you haven't taken the leap to start your own practice, start now. This could be a side hustle at a gym you go to. This could also be diving headfirst into doing this full time. You can't learn this stuff from the sideline. You have to be in the game.

- Get very clear on who your perfect customer is. Reference chapters 11 and 12 to help you with this.

- See business for what it is, a game. Think of the phases of this business as different belts you can achieve. Having no specific and attainable goal can create frustration and hurt your confidence. If you're at phase 1 of your cash practice right now, the goal is not to get to phase 5, it's to get to phase 2. You can't skip belts in Jiu Jitsu, and you can't skip phases in the game of business either.

- Learn to sell, and work on becoming a better storyteller. Use the patient journey framework I laid out in chapter 23. Stories help you connect with people, and it will make selling become much easier for you.

- Go change the world and have a major impact on all the people you can help in your business.

I hope you feel this book has been a great investment for your time. I've tried to put together a book that gives you the best possible chance of success in a cash-based Performance PT setting. No matter how helpful this book may be, it won't be as impactful as working with me or my team directly. If you'd like to work more closely with us, I highly recommend you take a look at www.physicaltherapybiz. com.

We have digital courses specifically designed to help you do things like start your business and get more new patients.

If you're looking for a unique group to be part of, I highly recommend taking a look at our PT Entrepreneur Mastermind. This is a one-of-a-kind opportunity to spend a couple days each year with me and my entire team. Not only that, but you get to be around an amazing group of successful Performance PTs. There is no better place for a PT entrepreneur than this group.

At these mastermind events, we spend a couple days diving deep into how to improve your business. This focuses on four key areas: people, processes, sales, marketing. We also have fun. We train together, we throw footballs at bowling pins together, and we get to know each other on a much more personal level. These people will become your network and help you get where you're trying to go in business.

Now that we're wrapping up this book, I want to leave you with a final message.

If you're like I was, sitting in my car not wanting to go to work, you have options. You can decide to do things differently now. You can go out on your own and set your own rules for how you work with patients. You don't have to be tied down by what insurance says you can and can't do.

It's happening all over the country. I see it every day in the people we work with. You're in the middle of a Performance PT revolution: A group of people who can function in the gray area between rehab and performance. A group of people who can have a long-term positive impact on people's health and wellness. A group of people who wake up every morning and love what they do for a living.

If you want to be one of these unique PTs, you can be. If you're already one, it's up to you to create an environment where you can fully use your skill set. This isn't a short sprint. This is a marathon, and consistency is what matters the most.

Don't read this book, freak out for a couple days, and then go back to whatever it is you've been doing.

Take action. Implement and follow through on the things you're trying to achieve.

We are so fortunate. We are among the lucky few people in this world who actually love what they do for a living. We would do it for free if we didn't have a mortgage and kids to buy food for. We just love helping other people, and we enjoy the process. There are millions of people out there right now driving to work and feeling depressed because they hate their job. If you function in the role of a Performance PT Entrepreneur, that will never be you.

Thanks for spending this time with me. I'll talk to you soon.
Danny Matta

ABOUT THE AUTHOR

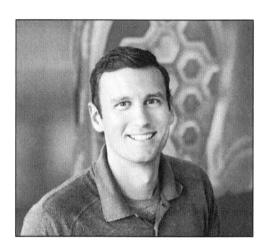

Danny Matta a former Army Physical Therapist turned entrepreneur. One fateful morning, he sat in his car questioning if he wanted to be a PT anymore. Burned out by an incredibly high volume of patients and endless documentation, he decided to leave his career as a PT in the Army. Knowing nothing about business, he dove headfirst into starting a cash-based PT clinic in a windowless room in the corner of a CrossFit gym. It worked out: Today, Matta not only serves his dream clients, he sees incredible revenue, employs a happy team of fellow PTs and enjoys the freedom of which he once only dreamed. He resides in Atlanta, GA his wife Ashley—the rock of the family—and their two crazy kids, Jack and Maggie.

Made in the USA
Middletown, DE
24 March 2019